EVALUATION OF CESAREAN DELIVERY

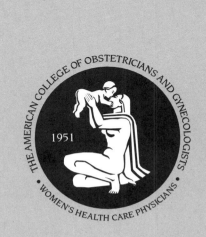

The American College of
Obstetricians and Gynecologists
Women's Health Care Physicians

409 12th Street, SW • PO Box 96920 • Washington, DC 20090-6920

Evaluation of Cesarean Delivery was developed under the direction of the Task Force on Cesarean Delivery Rates:

Roger K. Freeman, MD, Chair

Arnold W. Cohen, MD

Richard Depp III, MD

Fredric D. Frigoletto Jr, MD

Gary D.V. Hankins, MD

Ellice Lieberman, MD, DrPH

M. Kathryn Menard, MD

David A. Nagey, MD

Carol W. Saffold, MD

Lisa Sams, RNC, MSN (former Manager of Practice Development with the Association of Women's Health, Obstetric and Neonatal Nurses)

ACOG Staff

Stanley Zinberg, MD, MS

Debra A. Hawks, MPH

Elizabeth Steele

Library of Congress Cataloging-in-Publication Data

American College of Obstetricians and Gynecologists. Task Force on Cesarean Delivery Rates.
 Evaluation of cesarean delivery / [developed under the direction of the Task Force on Cesarean Delivery Rates, Roger K. Freeman ... et al.].
   p. ; cm.
 Includes index.
 ISBN 0-915473-62-3 (pbk.)
   1. Cesarean section—United States. 2. Cesarean section—United States—Statistics. I. Freeman, Roger K., 1935- II. Title.
 [DNLM: 1. Cesarean Section—utilization. 2. Utilization Review—methods. WQ 430 A512e 2000]
 RG761 .A486 2000
 618.8'6—dc21
                                                                                    00-038042

The information in *Evaluation of Cesarean Delivery* should not be viewed as a body of rigid rules. The guidelines are general and intended to be adapted to many different situations, taking into account the needs and resources particular to the locality, the institution, or the type of practice. Variations and innovations that improve the quality of patient care are to be encouraged rather than restricted. The purpose of these guidelines will be well served if they provide a firm basis on which local norms may be built.

12345/43210

Contents

Executive Summary

The increase in cesarean delivery rates in the United States has concerned the American College of Obstetricians and Gynecologists (ACOG) and other interested organizations for the past few decades. In 1994, ACOG issued a policy statement on this topic, and in 1995, ACOG's Health Care Commission held a focus session to determine ways to review and reduce cesarean delivery rates. This focus session led to the appointment in 1997 of ACOG's Task Force on Cesarean Delivery Rates, which was convened to assess the factors that contribute to the cesarean delivery rate in the United States, review the various proposed methodologies by which to reduce these rates, and develop guidance material to be made available to members of ACOG and other concerned institutions. This document, which is the work of the task force, is designed to assist institutions and individual practitioners in assessing, and if appropriate, reducing their cesarean delivery rates.

The factors that have contributed to the increased cesarean delivery rate in the United States during the past 25 years are not completely understood. This report will present evidence to show a wide variation in cesarean delivery rates between practitioners, hospitals, and geographic regions of the United States. In addition, nonmedical characteristics of patients, including payer type, socioeconomic status, ethnicity, and education are associated with significant variations in cesarean delivery rates. Aspects of physician practice, including solo versus group practice, employment status, in-house coverage, and education, also appear to be associated with variations in cesarean delivery rates. Finally, there is evidence that obstetric nursing plays a significant role in cesarean delivery rates.

When the variations in primary cesarean delivery rates are examined using patient characteristics, the highest variation occurs among nulliparous patients with term singleton fetuses with vertex presentations without other complications. High-risk patients have much lower variations in cesarean delivery rates between practitioners and hospitals. Differences in patient characteristics probably account for some of the variations in cesarean delivery rates and explain some of the differences between practitioners and hospitals. However, it appears that the most dramatic variations in primary cesarean delivery rates are found in nulliparous patients with normal term singleton fetuses with vertex presentations. Furthermore, it is not apparent that higher cesarean delivery rates in these lower-risk patients result in improved outcomes. Accordingly, it would seem appropriate to focus on low-risk nulliparous patients with term singleton fetuses with vertex presentations when evaluating strategies for lowering the primary cesarean delivery rate.

Patients with prior cesarean deliveries also have dramatic variations in rates of offered trial of labor and successful trial of labor. The variations associated with practitioner and nonpatient variables noted previously also apply to women who have had one prior cesarean delivery.

For analytic purposes, ACOG's Task Force on Cesarean Delivery Rates recommends using case-mix adjusted (normalized) cesarean delivery rates in patients who are 1) nulliparous with singleton term fetuses with vertex presentations, and 2) multiparous with one previous low-transverse cesarean delivery and term singleton fetuses with vertex presentations. Because these two groups of patients account for two thirds of all cesarean deliveries performed in the United States, they account for the greatest variations in cesarean delivery rates among practitioners, hospitals, and regions, thus providing an excellent opportunity to reduce cesarean delivery rates. Use of this case-mix adjusted approach should minimize confounding factors when comparing rates. Once case-mix adjusted cesarean delivery rates are available, cesarean delivery rate variations will be more meaningful and will allow for a more appropriate evaluation of practitioners' cesarean delivery rates. Outside benchmarks also will be helpful when comparing case-mix adjusted rates between practitioners.

The Healthy People 2000 Work Group recommended a target national cesarean delivery rate of 15% for the year 2000 (including the specific targets of 12% for primary [first time] cesarean deliveries and 65% for repeat cesarean deliveries among women who had a previous cesarean delivery); it is evident that this goal will not be met. A Department of Health and Human Services expert working group on cesarean delivery rates, which included ACOG representatives, discussed the *Healthy People 2010* objectives and developed evidence-based cesarean delivery rate goals for the year 2010. The National Center for Health Statistics (NCHS) has determined the cesarean delivery rates for two major categories of patients from 1996 birth certificate data. Target cesarean delivery rates determined by the expert working group were based on the 25th or 75th percentiles of state ranking of state rates for these two categories. Targets for the two major categories should be set at the 25th percentile for primary cesarean delivery rates and the 75th percentile for vaginal birth after cesarean delivery (VBAC) rates. The task force has adopted 1996 rates to be consistent with NCHS and the expert working group rates, but uses 1997 national vital statistics elsewhere in this report.

The expert working group proposes the following cesarean delivery rate benchmarks:

1. Nulliparous women at 37 weeks of gestation or greater with singleton fetuses with vertex presentations: The national 1996 cesarean delivery rate for this group was 17.9%; the expert working group goal at the 25th percentile for this group is 15.5%.

2. Multiparous women with one prior low-transverse cesarean delivery at 37 weeks of gestation or greater with singleton fetuses with

vertex presentations: The national 1996 VBAC rate for this group was 30.3%; the expert working group goal at the 75th percentile is 37%.

The task force also reviewed the risks associated with vaginal delivery, and identified long-term morbidity from pelvic floor injury associated with large fetuses, a prolonged second stage of labor, forceps delivery, midline episiotomies, and sphincter lacerations as concerns. Further research in these areas is recommended before practice guidelines can be made. The task force also recognized that risks associated with VBAC, particularly the potential risk of uterine rupture and its consequences to the mother and fetus, may have increased with relaxation of the indications and criteria used for selecting patients to be offered a trial of labor. Further research regarding attempted VBAC in patients with multifetal gestation, fetal macrosomia, or more than one prior cesarean delivery, as well as external cephalic version in women who have had a prior cesarean birth, is indicated.

Although cesarean delivery rate analysis may help obstetric institutions and practitioners adjust their practice patterns, cesarean delivery rates alone are not an indicator of quality. All practitioners have some patients in their practices who are at increased risk for cesarean delivery, regardless of management practices. Therefore, it is inappropriate to use unadjusted cesarean delivery rates to assess individual institutions or obstetric practitioners. Cesarean delivery rates that have not been adjusted for case mix have limited value.

It is hoped that the development of an approach using case-mix adjusted cesarean delivery rates with outside benchmarks for comparison will be a useful tool for practitioners, hospitals, health plans, and regional medical services. These entities are encouraged to focus on areas where cesarean delivery rates can be lowered while improving quality of care.

Modes of Delivery

What Are the Risks Associated with Cesarean Delivery?

Maternal Risks

Maternal mortality attributed to cesarean delivery is difficult to calculate, because the incidence of maternal death sometimes is due to underlying disease rather than the surgical procedure. Data indicate that the maternal mortality rate associated with cesarean delivery is 3–7 times greater than that associated with vaginal delivery (1). The overall mortality rate from cesarean delivery alone is 6 per 100,000 procedures (2).

Many authors have studied potential intraoperative and postoperative complications associated with cesarean delivery (1, 3–5). Intraoperatively, uterine hemorrhage may develop from atony, extension of the incision, uterine rupture, the presence of leiomyomata, or placenta accreta (4). Involvement of adjacent structures may occur in the form of urinary tract injury, which may include cystotomy or ureteral injury. Vaginal or broad ligament extension of the lower-segment uterine incision increases the risk of ureteral involvement.

Injuries to the gastrointestinal tract are rare and are estimated to occur in 1 in 1,300 cesarean deliveries (6). The history of previous infection or surgery, which may cause intraperitoneal adhesions, increases the risk of enterotomy.

In a study of catastrophic complications, 2.4% of patients with a prior cesarean delivery were found to have an extremely serious complication, including uterine rupture, placenta previa or accreta, and maternal or fetal death (7, 8). The leading causes of maternal mortality associated with cesarean delivery are deep vein thrombosis and pulmonary embolism.

Infection is the most common postoperative sequela of cesarean delivery. The observed incidence of endomyometritis varies greatly, with estimates ranging from 10% to 50%, compared with 1–3% of vaginal deliveries (9). Factors that contribute to this infection rate include the length of labor and rupture of membranes, the number of vaginal examinations, the use of internal monitors, and the patient's socioeconomic status (3, 10). In addition, the presence of chorioamnionitis and the duration of the surgical procedure may influence the rate of endomyometritis (11). Maternal factors of obesity and diabetes mellitus also may increase the risk of infection (10). Other, less frequent postoperative complications include wound and urinary tract infections, ileus, and atelectasis.

Multiple studies have highlighted the important association between previous cesarean delivery and placenta previa (12–17). The frequency of placenta previa in women who previously delivered vaginally is estimated at 0.3% (14, 15). A recent meta-analysis demonstrated that women with at least one prior cesarean delivery were 2.6 times more likely to develop placenta previa in a subsequent pregnancy (12). Other studies have shown that this risk increases with each subsequent cesarean birth (14).

Placenta accreta occurs frequently in patients with placenta previa and previous uterine scars. Patients without uterine scars face only a 4.5% risk of accreta (18, 19) versus an estimated risk from 24% (14) to 38% (18) in patients with placenta previa and uterine scars. When placenta accreta occurs, the patient faces the risk of massive hemorrhage and emergency peripartum hysterectomy. The fact that the risk of placenta accreta, a potentially life-threatening condition, increases with cesarean delivery further supports the need to reduce the cesarean delivery rate (14). If the cesarean delivery rate continues to remain high, institutions must be prepared to manage the potential complication of severe hemorrhage associated with higher rates of placenta accreta (8, 20).

Neonatal Risks

The mortality rate of infants delivered by cesarean birth in 1997 was 10.1 per 1,000 deliveries (21). This rate may be partly accounted for by risk factors that led to the cesarean birth, as well as inappropriate timing of delivery in some cases. Iatrogenic prematurity may be prevented by adhering to accurate pregnancy dating parameters. In addition to respiratory distress syndrome, elective surgical delivery without labor may contribute to transient tachypnea of the newborn, a condition that often requires intensive care treatment (22). Lastly, approximately 0.4% of infants delivered by cesarean birth experience accidental lacerations (22).

What Are the Risks Associated with Vaginal Delivery?

Vaginal delivery has risks similar to cesarean delivery (eg, deep vein thrombosis and pulmonary emboli) although they occur less frequently. As the obstetric community develops strategies to reduce the cesarean delivery rate, the number of spontaneous and operative vaginal deliveries will increase. In this regard, it is important to examine the implications that such an increase in vaginal deliveries may have on the incidence of pelvic floor dysfunction. Expanding clinical evidence shows that childbirth trauma resulting from vaginal delivery is a major factor in the development of pelvic floor dysfunctions such as fecal and urinary incontinence.

One study identified several causes of injury to the pelvic floor (23). Direct compression in the midpelvis from fetal head descent and stretching of pelvic structures and pudendal nerves during the second stage of labor may contribute to pelvic floor injuries. In addition, distension during the delivery of the head and shoulders through the pelvic diaphragm may traumatize the levator ani muscle (24). Mediolateral episiotomy has been shown to decrease pelvic floor strength by damaging the levator ani. Midline episiotomy subjects the patient to a greater risk of external anal sphincter rupture.

Several studies comparing parous women with nulliparous controls demonstrated that vaginal deliv-

ery also causes quantitative and qualitative changes in the pelvic floor that compromise the continence mechanisms (25–27). These changes include a lower vesical neck position at rest, hypermobility of the bladder neck during Valsalva's maneuver, and a decreased ability to elevate the vesical neck during pelvic contraction (25). One study also observed that vaginal delivery is associated with a lowered perineal position at rest, greater descent of the perineum during straining, an increased threshold of anal mucosa sensitivity, and increased bilateral pudendal nerve terminal motor latency (PNTML) (26).

Researchers have studied damage to the innervation of the pelvic floor musculature by comparing the change in PNTML in patients who had cesarean deliveries and vaginal deliveries (28). Whereas vaginal delivery increased PNTML with risk factors for nerve damage, including multiparity, forceps delivery, a prolonged second stage of labor, third-degree lacerations, and fetal macrosomia, no change in pudendal nerve function was noted with cesarean delivery using epidural anesthesia. However, the pudendal nerve damage was reversible in 60% of patients who had vaginal deliveries when measurements were repeated 2 months postpartum. A later study demonstrated that macrosomia and a prolonged second stage of labor cause a significant prolongation of PNTML (29). Again, in elective cesarean delivery, no change in PNTML was observed. Cesarean delivery after labor showed a unilateral prolongation of PNTML. Although there are compelling data from prospective investigational studies, all are characterized by small sample sizes (122, 202, and 128 subjects) (28–30).

One study investigated the incidence of anal incontinence and anal sphincter rupture endosonographically in women who were nulliparous, multiparous, and had undergone cesarean delivery (30). Anal incontinence was symptomatic at 6 weeks postdelivery in 13% of nulliparous women and 23% of multiparous women. This study also showed a high incidence of asymptomatic anal sphincter defects diagnosed by ultrasonography; 35% of nulliparous women and 44% of multiparous women had anal sphincter defects at 6 weeks and 6 months postdelivery. In patients who had forceps deliveries, 80% showed anal sphincter defects compared with patients who had vacuum delivery who showed no defects.

Multiple studies report that vaginal delivery with third-degree laceration (partial or complete anal sphincter rupture) results in anal incontinence (31–36). Factors that increase the risk for anal sphincter trauma include use of forceps, a birth weight greater than 4 kg, occiput posterior fetal position, nulliparity, and midline episiotomy. Few long-term studies exist, but it appears that both anal and urinary incontinence symptoms persist or increase with maternal age (37).

The preponderance of published information on the effect of vaginal delivery on urinary function is derived from retrospective patient questionnaires and telephone interviews (38–41). The incidence of stress urinary incontinence was found to be 24.5% at 3 months after vaginal delivery, and 5.2% after cesarean delivery (38). In another study, the overall incidence of stress urinary incontinence in patients who had vaginal deliveries and episiotomies or spontaneous tears was approximately 36% (40).

Episiotomy was not found to protect against the development of stress urinary incontinence (40).

Current research on pelvic floor injury from vaginal delivery does not offer sufficient evidence to mandate a change in standard clinical management of labor and birth. Studies suggest, however, that patients who are at high risk of compromising their reconstructed normal pelvic floor following surgery for anal incontinence, urinary incontinence, and genital prolapse after vaginal delivery should be offered an elective cesarean delivery (42).

The prevalence of pelvic floor dysfunction after vaginal delivery suggests that obstetricians and other obstetric practitioners might assume a more active role in preventing pelvic floor trauma (23). Specific recommendations mentioned in the literature include minimizing the use of forceps and midline episiotomy, which increase the risk of anal sphincter rupture.

Nonobstetric Factors that Contribute to Variations in Cesarean Delivery Rates

There are many variations in cesarean delivery rates. Numerous factors—medical and nonmedical, actual and perceived—affect these rates, which provide ways to decrease the cesarean delivery rate.

The rates of cesarean deliveries vary greatly among institutions, geographic regions, and obstetric practitioners. These variations cannot be explained entirely by differences in medical or obstetric factors. Nonclinical factors such as practice culture, practice style, hospital environment, and source of payment also affect cesarean delivery rates. In order to develop a nationwide approach to provide patients with the appropriate delivery based on medical and obstetric considerations, variations in nonclinical factors that influence the method of delivery must first be understood and evaluated.

What Are the Implications of Variation in Cesarean Delivery Rates by Region?

There is wide variation in cesarean delivery rates among regions in the United States, as well as among states within those regions. National data on cesarean delivery rates are available from two sources: 1) live birth certificates (43, 44), and 2) the National Hospital Discharge Survey (NHDS) (45, 46). The NHDS rates are estimated from a sample of 27,000 women who were discharged after giving birth from short-stay, nonfederal hospitals participating in the NHDS.

The states with higher cesarean delivery rates are clustered in the southern and northeastern regions, while rates tend to be lower in the western and midwestern states (Fig. 1). This general trend has been fairly consistent over time (Table 1).

According to 1997 national vital statistics reports, state cesarean delivery rates ranged from a high of 26.7 in Mississippi to a low of 15.3 in Colorado (44). Total cesarean delivery rates tend to parallel primary cesarean delivery rates. Generally, states with low cesarean delivery rates have high VBAC rates, but there is substantial variation. Reported VBAC rates in 1997 ranged from 44.7 to 13.0 (Fig. 2) (44).

Although data indicate that regional variations in cesarean delivery rates do exist in the United States, little has been published on factors contributing to these variations. Similar regional patterns were noted when rates were adjusted for differences between states in maternal age and birth order distribution (45). Cesarean delivery rates by race are generally similar within regions, with the exception of the West (Table 2). African-American women in the West have a higher rate of total cesarean delivery and a lower rate of VBAC than non-Hispanic white and Hispanic women. Other factors known to be associated with variation in cesarean delivery rates, such as insurance status, education, type of hospital, and maternal weight gain, have not been investigated in the context of regional variation.

There is also very little information in the literature regarding variation in cesarean delivery rates in urban versus nonurban settings. However, one investigation, using 1987 birth certificate data from Washington State, calculated similar hospital-specific cesarean birth rates for urban and nonurban settings (47). Wide variation in cesarean delivery rates by state and region suggests an opportunity for improvement.

■ RECOMMENDATION

- Researchers should study the factors contributing to regional variations in cesarean delivery rates, in order to guide effective intervention.

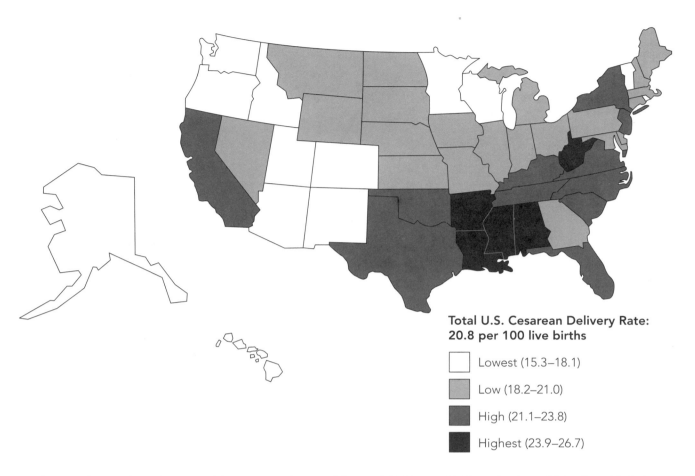

Total U.S. Cesarean Delivery Rate: 20.8 per 100 live births

☐ Lowest (15.3–18.1)

▨ Low (18.2–21.0)

▨ High (21.1–23.8)

■ Highest (23.9–26.7)

■ **Figure 1.** State ranking of cesarean delivery rates in the United States, 1997. (Ventura SJ, Martin JA, Curtin SC, Mathews TJ. Births: final data for 1997. Natl Vital Stat Rep 1999;47:1–84)

Is Hospital Volume a Factor?

Although there is a perception that hospital volume influences cesarean delivery rates, this relationship, if it exists, is not always consistent. Recent data from the NHDS suggest that there is no clear relationship between hospital volume and cesarean birth rates (46, 48). However, these data are not case-mix adjusted. It is conceivable that hospitals with higher volumes care for more high-risk women. Thus, adjusting for case mix might potentially uncover important differences in cesarean delivery rates. Variations in VBAC rates by hospital volume also warrant more attention.

Are Teaching Versus Nonteaching Hospitals a Factor?

Cesarean delivery rates are lower in teaching and county hospitals. This may be due to improved supervision as well as compliance with clinical management protocols for common indications based on the hospital's training mission (49–52).

How Do Practitioner Characteristics Affect the Cesarean Delivery Rate?

What Is the Role of 24-Hour Obstetric Coverage?

Local hospital environment and culture also appear to influence cesarean delivery rates. Hospitals that provide 24-hour, dedicated in-house physician coverage show lower cesarean delivery rates (51, 53, 54). One study showed a reduced cesarean delivery rate when there was a full-time, in-house obstetrician present, compared with the cesarean delivery rates prior to in-house coverage and compared with

Table 1. Rates of Cesarean Delivery and Vaginal Birth After Cesarean Delivery by Region: United States, 1989, 1993, 1995, and 1997

Region	Total Cesarean Delivery Rates				Primary Cesarean Delivery Rates	Vaginal Birth After Cesarean Delivery Rates	
	1989	1993	1995	1997	1997	1995	1997
United States	22.8	21.8	20.8	20.8	14.6	27.5	27.4
Northeast	23.8	22.5	21.5	20.1	15.6	31.4	33.8
Midwest	22.1	20.4	19.3	18.9	13.3	30.3	30.5
South	24.8	23.8	22.8	22.7	15.9	23.9	23.5
West	21.2	19.7	19.1	17.5	13.3	27.0	33.0

Clarke SC, Taffel SM. State variations in rates of cesarean and VBAC delivery: 1989 and 1993. Stat Bull Metrop Insur Co 1996;77:28–36

physicians who did not adopt full-time in-house obstetric physician coverage (54).

■ CONCLUSION

- In hospitals and practitioner groups with high cesarean delivery rates, the provision of dedicated 24-hour, in-house obstetric coverage has been beneficial in reducing cesarean deliveries in some of these groups.

How Is Practitioner Style Related to Cesarean Delivery?

There appears to be a pattern of clinical behavior associated with practice style (55, 56). Cesarean delivery rates are higher for male obstetricians and board-certified obstetricians (57). Patterns of nursing care provided to laboring patients also appear to be related to the cesarean delivery rate (see also "How Does Intrapartum Nursing Affect the Cesarean Delivery Rate?") (58). There are weak data to link cesarean delivery rates with medical–legal fears and practitioner leisure time (59–61).

Are Differences in Payer Source Associated with the Cesarean Delivery Rate?

Studies report that cesarean delivery rates often are related to the source of payment. Rather, women who have private medical insurance are more likely to have a cesarean delivery than those insured by a health maintenance organization or by public insurance (49, 50, 62–71). Cesarean delivery rates vary from as high as 29.1% in patients with private medical insurance to 15.6% in patients who are indigent (67).

Source of payment not only affects the total cesarean delivery rate, but VBAC rates as well (65, 67). The cesarean delivery rate also varies according to race, because it has been found that Hispanic and Asian women have lower cesarean delivery rates than African–American women, who in turn have lower rates than Caucasian women (50) (Table 2).

■ RECOMMENDATIONS

- Hospitals should evaluate variations in cesarean delivery rates among practitioners at their institution.

- The obstetric community should educate clinicians, hospital management, and patients that cesarean delivery based on nonclinical factors (eg, solo practitioners, group staff model, teaching hospital, payment source) is not associated with improved maternal or neonatal outcomes.

- Institutions should use comparative outside data on cesarean delivery rates to evaluate their own cesarean delivery rates.

- Hospitals or practitioner groups with high cesarean delivery rates can consider establishing separate 24-hour, in-house obstetric coverage by physicians who are solely responsible for the management of the intrapartum patient.

How Does Intrapartum Nursing Affect the Cesarean Delivery Rate?

Strategies to reduce the cesarean delivery rate in the United States have focused primarily on efforts to alter physician practice. However, the interdisciplinary nature of care for a woman in labor should be

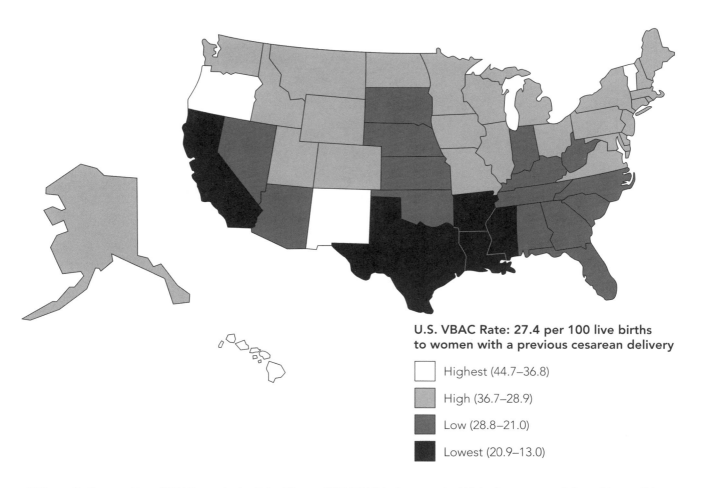

U.S. VBAC Rate: 27.4 per 100 live births to women with a previous cesarean delivery

☐ Highest (44.7–36.8)

▨ High (36.7–28.9)

▨ Low (28.8–21.0)

■ Lowest (20.9–13.0)

■ **Figure 2.** State ranking of VBAC rates in the United States, 1997. VBAC indicates vaginal birth after cesarean delivery. (Ventura SJ, Martin JA, Curtin SC, Mathews TJ. Births: final data for 1997. Natl Vital Stat Rep 1999;47:1–84)

considered. Some studies have shown variations in nurses' cesarean delivery rates that may have a positive or negative impact (72). Although an interesting concept, little attention has thus far been given to studying the effect of intrapartum nursing care on the cesarean delivery rate. Yet, the systematic review of several studies related to the care of women in labor indicate that the presence of a trained individual who provides comfort measures and support does affect patient outcome.

In addition, one study indicates that the continuous care and monitoring that the intrapartum nurse provides to the woman throughout her labor appears to bear some relation to the cesarean delivery rate. This study examined the influence of nursing care by statistically evaluating the cesarean delivery rate for nurses who provided care to healthy nulliparous women with term singleton pregnancies (58). The study found that the cesarean delivery rate for individual nurses ranged from 4.9% to 19%. This wide range could not be explained by differences in maternal age and gravity, attendance of mother at childbirth class, insurance status, reliance on public assistance, attending physician, use of epidural anesthesia, augmentation of labor, dilatation when the nurse assumed care, infant weight, or gestational age.

However, the amount of time that labor nurses spend with the patient, especially regarding comforting measures and reassurance may be limited. Two work sampling studies examined the amount of time the intrapartum nurse spends providing comfort measures and support to the woman in labor (73, 76). Nursing care activities were divided into two groups, direct and indirect care, with supportive direct care activities measured in four categories. Both studies show that nurses spent less than 10% of the time (6.1% [76] and 9.9% [73]) providing supportive care to women. In fact, 74.9% of the nurses' time was spent

Table 2. Rates of Cesarean Delivery and of Vaginal Birth After Cesarean Delivery by Race of Mother: United States, 1997

Region	Total Cesarean Rate*				Primary Cesarean Rate†				Vaginal Birth After Previous Cesarean Rate‡			
	All Races	Non-Hispanic White	Non-Hispanic Black	Hispanic	All Races	Non-Hispanic White	Non-Hispanic Black	Hispanic	All Races	Non-Hispanic White	Non-Hispanic Black	Hispanic
Northeast	20.1	20.4	21.1	19.1	15.6	15.5	16.5	15.1	33.8	33.8	33.1	32.2
Midwest	18.9	19.2	18.4	18.5	13.3	13.5	13.2	11.8	30.5	30.5	31.8	32.0
South	22.7	23.0	23.1	19.4	15.9	16.2	16.3	14.5	23.5	23.1	24.3	28.6
West	17.5	18.1	21.1	17.6	13.3	13.6	15.5	12.6	33.0	32.1	29.6	33.3

* Percent of all births by cesarean delivery.
† Primary cesarean deliveries per 100 live births to women who have not had a previous cesarean delivery.
‡ Vaginal births after previous cesarean delivery per 100 live births to women with a previous cesarean delivery.
Data from Ventura SJ, Martin JA, Curtin SC, Mathews TJ. Births: final data for 1997. Natl Vital Stat Rep 1999;47:1–84

apart from women in labor, over half of which (47.6%) was spent completing tasks such as charting, patient reporting, or preparing drugs and equipment (76).

In contrast, there are suggestions that women may benefit from direct comfort and support measures provided during labor (75, 76). One randomized trial compared one-to-one nursing care with usual care and found no effect on cesarean delivery rates (76), although there was a 17% risk reduction for oxytocin in the study group. A randomized controlled trial failed to reproduce these results (75).

A meta-analysis of nonrandomized studies (primarily in developing countries) showed significant reductions in cesarean delivery rates in association with the provision of a support person to women in labor (77). The Cochrane analysis further indicates that women who received this support had shorter labor, were less likely to need intrapartum analgesia, anesthesia, or an operative vaginal delivery. Also, it was less likely that their newborn's 5-minute Apgar scores would be less than 7 (79). In addition, the Cochrane analysis shows a decreased cesarean delivery rate in settings where women were not allowed to have a family member present but did have a support person. Despite the variation in training for the support person, Cochrane reports consistency in the experimental intervention with the continuous presence of the support person who offers comforting touch and verbal encouragement (79).

In contrast to the evidence that comfort measures and support affect outcome, there are little data to show that intrapartum nurses incorporate these techniques in daily care or that clinical education and training programs include this evidence. Furthermore, the emphasis on technology in intrapartum care and the significant limitation of nursing time are seen as potential barriers to the application of this evidence in practice (79). Appendix A contains a form that obstetric institutions can use to track the nursing services provided to women in labor.

■ CONCLUSION

- The continuous presence of a trained individual who provides comfort and support to women in labor may lead to lower cesarean delivery rates in some patient populations, and a reduction in medical interventions.

■ STRATEGIES

- Institutions with high cesarean delivery rates should review nurses' direct and indirect care responsibilities.
- Institutions with high cesarean delivery rates should review individual cesarean delivery rates for nurses, similarly to physician-specific rates.

■ RECOMMENDATION

- Researchers should further study the value of labor support and other possible nursing interventions, and the means whereby they may act on cesarean delivery rates.

Does Fear of Litigation Affect the Cesarean Delivery Rate?

Before 1970, litigation for poor fetal outcome was rare. At that time, only auscultation and observation for meconium were used to assess fetal well-being during labor. Before transfusions and antibiotics became readily available, the maternal risks of hemorrhage and infection associated with cesarean delivery were far too great to justify cesarean delivery for fetal indications. As a result, success was declared even if a difficult forceps birth resulted in a depressed fetus and damage to the maternal tissues, and failure was declared if cesarean delivery was the final resort.

With the advent of electronic fetal monitoring (EFM), improved neonatal care, and improved measures for maternal safety, cesarean delivery became more acceptable. This was due mainly to the common belief that most cases of cerebral palsy were the result of intrapartum asphyxia or vaginal delivery trauma. Consequently, increased EFM and the decreased number of forceps deliveries led to an increase in the cesarean delivery rate for fetal indications and an expectation for optimal outcome. It was believed by most obstetricians that avoiding asphyxia and mechanical birth trauma through cesarean delivery would markedly decrease the incidence of cerebral palsy and mental retardation. Conversely, studies have shown that despite an exponential increase in EFM and cesarean deliveries, and a near disappearance of forceps and vaginal breech deliveries in some cases, the incidence of cerebral palsy remains unchanged (80). Critical assessment of long-term outcomes in the National Collaborative Perinatal Project (NCCP) also has shown that only a small minority of cases of cerebral palsy can be attributed to intrapartum events (81).

The significance of these recent findings has increased after a groundswell of litigation based on the premise that virtually all cases of intrapartum fetal death or subsequent cerebral palsy were preventable by the obstetrician. Even so, the gradual dissemination of data from the NCCP as well as criteria for causation of neurologic damage published by ACOG (82) and the American Academy of Pediatrics has had little apparent impact on changing obstetric behavior or in preventing the continued excess of litigation for bad neurologic outcomes unrelated to intrapartum events. In fact, one study estimated that approximately 25% of cesarean deliveries are performed for medical–legal concerns (83). Another study showed that 84% of U.S. obstetricians polled perceived the threat of medical litigation to be the leading reason for the increase in cesarean deliveries (84). Other studies have shown that higher medical liability insurance premiums also are associated with higher cesarean delivery rates (85, 86). The fact that most obstetricians have been sued for medical malpractice at least once (87), has only added to the perception that, when in doubt, cesarean delivery is good, defensive medicine.

Although data to support the threat of litigation are weak, the perceived threat of litigation continues to influence obstetric behavior regarding cesarean delivery. Perhaps this trend could be reversed if initiatives were taken, such as those in California, to implement tort reform to reduce the number of malpractice lawsuits and medical liability insurance premiums.

■ Conclusions

- Reform of medical liability laws and legal procedures may reduce the cesarean delivery rate.
- Education of physicians, nurses, attorneys, and the public regarding the causation of perinatal brain damage may assist in reducing unwarranted litigation.

■ STRATEGY

The obstetric community should educate physicians, nurses, attorneys, and the public regarding the actual relationship between brain damage and perinatal events; this may reduce unwarranted litigation.

■ Recommendation

- The obstetric community should seek reform of medical liability laws and legal procedures, which may result in reducing the cesarean delivery rate.

Maternal Characteristics

Is Maternal Age a Risk Factor for Cesarean Delivery?

In 1970, only 4% of first births were to women older than 30 years. By 1986, that percentage had more than tripled to 14.8% (85). By 1994, 21% of first births were to women older than 30 years, and 5.8% were to women older than 35 years.

Studies have consistently found a higher rate of cesarean delivery for both nulliparous and multiparous women at least 35 years of age (89–106). For nulliparous women in this age group, studies performed in the United States almost uniformly have reported an approximate twofold higher risk of cesarean delivery (92, 93, 96–103). Studies performed in other countries often have reported higher relative risks, possibly related to a higher rate of elective cesarean delivery and induction of labor, with maternal age being the primary indication (91, 100, 105). Women at least 40 years of age at the time of their first delivery may be at an even slightly higher risk (101, 104). Although the absolute rate of cesarean delivery is lower among multiparous women, older multiparous women giving birth also have been reported to be at about twice the risk of having a cesarean delivery than their younger counterparts (93, 94, 96, 100–102). Some studies have reported increases in cesarean deliveries both for failure to progress and for nonreassuring fetal status, suggesting that the higher rate of cesarean deliveries among older women is not related to any specific indication (94, 103).

Studies examining the cesarean delivery rate across the entire reproductive age spectrum have noted a continuous increase in the cesarean delivery rate from the youngest to the oldest groups of women giving birth (94, 101). Although it has been suggested that adolescents may be at an increased risk for cesarean delivery, one meta-analysis indicated that in developed countries adolescents actually are at lower risk for cesarean delivery (107).

The reason for the increase in cesarean deliveries among older women is not entirely clear. Although older women may be more likely to have other characteristics that increase their risk for cesarean delivery, such as higher rates of chronic medical conditions (93, 95, 96, 98) and higher rates of pregnancy and labor complications (91, 93, 96, 99, 101–105, 109) (reported in some but not all studies), studies examining the rate of cesarean delivery in subgroups of the population with uncomplicated pregnancies (93, 97) have still noted the association of age with cesarean delivery. However, no single study has taken into account all of the known confounding factors. For example, studies examining a subgroup with uncomplicated pregnancies have not taken into account whether labor was induced or spontaneous (93, 97). Induction has been reported to be a more frequent procedure in older women (91, 104, 105). The only study examining the association between age and cesarean delivery among women with spontaneous labor did not take into account the increased occurrence of medical complications (98).

In addition to the increased prevalence of medical risks, two other major interpretations have been proposed to explain the increase in cesarean deliveries among older women. One explanation is that practitioners' attitudes toward the pregnancies and labor of older women, particularly nulliparous women, contribute to the increased cesarean delivery rate in that group. One study, for example, noting a higher rate of primary elective cesarean delivery among older nulliparous and multiparous women, concluded that maternal age alone may influence a clinician's decision regarding cesarean delivery (104). The high social value placed on a birth to an older nulliparous woman, discussed since the earliest considerations of this issue, still resonates within the current literature (97). Despite studies indicating a positive outcome among older pregnant women (108, 110), it also has been suggested that practitioners' misperceptions about the risk status of older women may contribute to the increased rate (96, 97).

Alternatively, it has been suggested that the difference in cesarean delivery rates also may reflect differences in the labor of younger and older women (97). A number of studies have noted a higher rate of labor abnormalities among older women, including longer labor (96, 99), particularly in the second stage (95, 98, 99, 101, 102, 108), as well as more active phase arrest and arrest of descent (99). In some studies, this higher rate of cesarean delivery occurred despite an increased rate of oxytocin augmentation in the group of older women (96, 98, 102). One investigation, for instance, concluded that this persistence argues against the contention that practitioner attitude is the main reason for the increase, and supports the hypothesis of less effective uterine contractions in older women (98).

Taken together, the literature suggests that the higher rate of cesarean delivery among older women is based on a number of factors related to age. For example, older women are more likely to have chronic medical conditions and pregnancy complications. Though not extensive, some existing data also suggest that older women tend to have longer labor, are more often diagnosed with arrest disorders, and are less responsive to treatment with oxytocin. The literature additionally supports the theory that practitioners' attitudes toward pregnancy in older women also may contribute to the increase in the rate of cesarean deliveries, particularly among older nulliparous women for whom this may be their only pregnancy.

■ STRATEGY

- Obstetric practitioners should not perform cesarean delivery for the sole indication of maternal age.

■ RECOMMENDATION

- The obstetric community should study the relationship between maternal age and cesarean delivery.

Are Maternal Prepregnancy Weight and Weight Gain During Pregnancy Risk Factors for Cesarean Delivery?

Most studies conducted have noted a significant association between high maternal prepregnancy weight and an increased risk of cesarean delivery with rate ratios ranging from 1.2 to 2.8 (111–119). Several studies have separately examined the effects of both prepregnancy weight and weight gain during pregnancy as risk factors for cesarean birth (111, 112, 120). One study found a 16.3% cesarean delivery rate among women who gained more than 35 lb, compared with a 9.2% rate among women who gained less than that amount (RR=1.76, 95% CI=1.46, 2.13) (111). Another study found an increase of similar magnitude in the low-risk nulliparous population, with a cesarean delivery rate of 22.6% for those who gained at least 19.5 kg, compared with a 15.0% rate for those who gained less (RR=1.51, 95% CI=1.35, 1.69) (112). In multiple logistic regression analyses controlling for a variety of factors (including maternal height, age, and parity, as well as infant birth weight), both maternal prepregnancy body mass index (BMI [weight in kilograms divided by height in meters squared]) and maternal weight gain remained independent predictors of cesarean delivery (111, 120).

The best controlled studies suggest that there is a higher rate of cesarean delivery associated with both higher maternal prepregnancy weight and greater prenatal weight gain. The reasons for the association, however, are unclear. Although infant birth weight is higher among women who weigh more, the association between maternal weight and weight gain and cesarean birth persisted in multivariate analyses, even when birth weight was taken into account. In addition, although obese women more frequently have conditions such as diabetes and hypertension, which are associated with an increased risk of cesarean delivery, the association between obesity and cesarean delivery persists even when women with those conditions are excluded or when those factors are controlled in multivariate analyses (111, 112, 115). Although an increase in fetal heart rate abnormalities among obese women has been reported (111), other data suggest that anthropometric factors are more strongly associated with the use of cesarean delivery for maternal indications (such as failure to progress and medical complications) than for fetal indications (such as fetal distress and macrosomia) (112). It also has been suggested that the increase in cesarean deliveries in the presence of obesity may result from an increase in pelvic soft tissue that narrows the birth canal (115).

Over the past 25 years, changes in both the prevalence of women overweight prior to pregnancy and the amount of weight gained during pregnancy may have contributed to the increase in cesarean deliveries. National data from the early 1970s to the early 1990s indicate a substantial increase in the number of overweight women (defined as BMI≥ 27.3) of childbearing age (121). For women aged 20–29 years, the percentage increased from 12.6% to 20.2%; for women aged 30–39 years, the percentage increased from 22.9% to 34.3% (121). Data suggest that currently 40% of young adult women are obese (BMI>29) (118, 122). In addition, beginning in 1970, there was also a shift away from limiting weight gain during pregnancy (123). From the 1960s to the 1990s, the average weight gain during pregnancy increased from 22 to 33 lb, an increase of 50% (123), and the average infant birth weight increased by 111–150 g. Because of the increased risk of cesarean birth associated with higher weight gain, one study suggested a reevaluation of the new higher weight gain recommendations of the Institute of Medicine (111).

■ STRATEGY

- Obstetric practitioners should educate women about the direct association between prepregnancy weight and weight gain during pregnancy, and the risk of cesarean delivery.

■ RECOMMENDATION

- Current maternal weight gain recommendations should be reviewed to determine their contribution to cesarean delivery rates.

Obstetric and Medical Issues that Affect Cesarean Delivery Rates

Can Vaginal Delivery After Cesarean Delivery Reduce the Cesarean Delivery Rate?

In 1997, 37% of cesarean deliveries in the United States were repeat cesarean deliveries. In 1997, 27.4% of women who had a previous cesarean delivery had a subsequent successful vaginal delivery (44). Table 3 indicates how the total and primary cesarean delivery rates gradually decreased and the VBAC rate gradually increased from 1989 to 1997. The VBAC rate, as defined by ACOG, refers to the number of women delivering by VBAC divided by the total number of women bearing children after a previous cesarean delivery, times 100. The trial of labor rate, as defined by ACOG, refers to the number of women who undergo a trial of labor divided by the number of women considered to be eligible to be offered VBAC.

There is wide regional variation in the proportion of women who undergo VBAC (see Table 1). The 1997 U.S. VBAC rate of 27.4 is in sharp contrast to VBAC rates of European countries of approximately 50.0 (125).

There is strong consensus within the obstetric community that a trial of labor is appropriate for most women who have had a single previous low-transverse cesarean delivery, even though the procedure of trial of labor entails some degree of risk to both mother and fetus (124, 126). Despite 800 citations in the literature, there are no randomized trials to show that maternal and neonatal outcomes are better with VBAC than with repeat cesarean delivery. Published evidence, most of which emanates from tertiary care centers, suggests that the benefits of VBAC outweigh the risks in most women with a single prior low-transverse cesarean birth (124).

Published series indicate that 60–80% of VBAC candidates undergoing a trial of labor will deliver vaginally (127–129). Women who have undergone vaginal delivery at least once have a higher VBAC rate than women with a prior cesarean birth who have not delivered vaginally (130, 131). Similarly, women who had a cesarean delivery for a nonrecurring indication (eg, breech presentation) for their first delivery are more likely to have a successful vaginal delivery

Table 3. Total and Primary Cesarean Delivery Rates and Vaginal Birth after Previous Cesarean Delivery Rates: United States, 1989–1997

Year	Cesarean Delivery Rate		Vaginal Birth After Cesarean Delivery Rate‡
	Total*	Primary†	
1997	20.8	14.6	27.4
1996	20.7	14.6	28.3
1995	20.8	14.7	27.5
1994	21.2	14.9	26.3
1993	21.8	15.3	24.3
1992	22.3	15.6	22.6
1991	22.6	15.9	21.3
1990	22.7	16.0	19.9
1989	22.8	16.1	18.9

* Percent of all live births by cesarean delivery.

† Number of primary cesarean deliveries per 100 live births to women who have not had a previous cesarean delivery.

‡ Number of vaginal births after previous cesarean delivery per 100 live births to women with a previous cesarean delivery.

Ventura SJ, Martin JA, Curtin SC, Mathews TJ. Births: final data for 1997. Natl Vital Stat Rep 1999;47:1–84

17

(130). There is no completely reliable method to predict whether a trial of labor will be successful in an individual patient. Successful VBAC is associated with less morbidity than a repeat cesarean birth, but patients who undergo cesarean delivery after a trial of labor run a higher risk of infection and other maternal morbidity (124).

The most serious risk of VBAC is the potential for catastrophic uterine rupture, which can result in fetal anoxic injury or death. Based on available literature, the occurrence of uterine rupture in women with a single prior low-transverse cesarean delivery is 0.2–1.5% (124). The proportion of uterine ruptures that result in significant maternal and neonatal morbidity is difficult to glean from available literature (132). Cohort studies have not demonstrated differences in perinatal morbidity and mortality among infants of women who attempted a trial of labor after previous cesarean delivery compared with women who opted for repeat cesarean delivery (56, 133, 134). However, because uterine rupture is an uncommon event, these studies lack the power to detect potentially important differences. Reports of catastrophic uterine rupture appear as case reports or small-case series without the denominators necessary to calculate risk (135–137).

Rupture of the uterine scar can be life-threatening for both mother and infant (132, 135, 136, 139). When catastrophic uterine rupture occurs, some patients will require hysterectomy and some infants will die or will be neurologically impaired (134, 135). In most cases, the cause of uterine rupture in a patient who has undergone VBAC is unknown, but poor outcomes can result even in appropriate candidates with proper management.

When uterine rupture does occur, generally the outcome is good for mother and infant (126). The immediate availability of a physician throughout active labor who is capable of monitoring labor and performing an emergency cesarean delivery, as well as available anesthesia and personnel for an emergency cesarean delivery, is necessary (124).

The following list summarizes ACOG VBAC recommendations (124):

1. Most women with one previous cesarean delivery with a low-transverse incision are candidates for VBAC and should be counseled about VBAC and offered a trial of labor.

2. A previous uterine incision extending into the fundus is a contraindication for VBAC.

3. Because uterine rupture may be catastrophic, VBAC should be attempted in institutions equipped to respond to emergencies with physicians immediately available to provide emergency care.

The factors that influence a decision about whether to attempt a trial of labor after previous cesarean birth are poorly understood. Reports suggest that pregnant women play an important role in making the decision as to whether they should attempt VBAC. Given the option, 30–50% of them choose elective repeat cesarean delivery (139). The most frequent reasons given for this choice are fear of failed trial of labor, concerns about the dangers of vaginal birth, fear of pain, desire for sterilization, and convenience in scheduling. Studies have found that there are higher VBAC rates among younger practitioners in more specialized hospitals, and among patients with a lower level of education (139, 140).

There are several published, randomized studies of interventions designed to increase VBAC rates. One study in Ontario compared the impact of opinion leaders to the impact of audit with feedback. The cesarean delivery rate was reduced only in the group educated by the opinion leaders (71). A second Canadian study that focused on women's preferences tested the impact of a prenatal education and support program promoting VBAC. The investigators did not find a clinically significant increase in the rate of VBAC among women participating in the program (139). It should be noted, however, that the VBAC rate in this study was relatively high (at least 50%). Such a program might well be successful in areas with low VBAC rates. A number of cohort studies have documented that a VBAC program can be a safe and important component of hospital-based programs to reduce cesarean delivery (56, 136, 142, 143).

Repeat cesarean delivery accounts for more than one third of all cesarean deliveries in the United States and is the leading indication for cesarean birth. Wide variation in the practice of VBAC, however, suggests that clinician behavior may be susceptible to modification and therefore may play a role in reducing the repeat cesarean delivery rate. Table 4 depicts actual U.S. data from 1997 when the VBAC rate was 27.4 and the total cesarean delivery rate was 20.8. Varying the VBAC rate and holding the primary cesarean birth rate constant yields the change in total cesarean delivery rate depicted in the table. For example, if the VBAC rate had been 50.0, the total cesare-

Table 4. The Theoretic Impact of VBAC Rate on Total Cesarean Delivery Rate (Extrapolated from 1997 data)*

VBAC Rate	All Births	Total Births with Prior Cesarean Delivery	Primary Cesarean Deliveries	Total Cesarean Delivery	Repeat Cesarean Delivery	Total Vaginal Births After Cesarean Delivery	Total Cesarean Delivery Rate	Repeat Cesarean Delivery Rate
Projected impact of a reduced VBAC rate								
10.0				868,513	365,987	40,665	22.4	42.1
20.0				827,848	325,322	81,330	21.3	39.3
Actual 1997 data on cesarean deliveries								
27.4	3,880,894	406,652	502,526	797,033	294,507	112,145	20.8	37.0
Projected impact of an increased VBAC rate								
30.0				787,182	284,656	121,996	20.3	36.2
40.0				746,517	243,991	162,661	19.2	32.7
50.0				705,852	203,326	203,326	18.2	28.8
60.0				665,187	162,661	243,991	17.1	24.5

*Abbreviation: VBAC, vaginal birth after cesarean delivery.
Data from Ventura SJ, Martin JA, Curtin SC, Mathews TJ. Births: final data for 1997. Natl Vital Stat Rep 1999;47:1–84

an delivery rate in 1997 would have been 18.2. Further reduction in the total cesarean delivery rate would require a reduction in the primary cesarean delivery rate. There has been a substantial increase in the proportion of women with a prior cesarean delivery who undergo VBAC in recent years. However, the absolute number of repeat cesarean deliveries has not decreased, because the number of women with a primary uterine scar has increased (50).

The question remains as to what constitutes an appropriate VBAC rate. Established data sources such as vital records and hospital discharge data do not include the information required to estimate the number of candidates for a trial of labor who undergo elective repeat cesarean delivery. Some women are not candidates for a trial of labor because of a prior classical uterine incision. Others have contraindications to labor such as placenta previa, malpresentation, or a maternal or fetal condition. The proportion of women with a contraindication to trial of labor is likely to vary according to the characteristics of the patient population.

CONCLUSIONS

- VBAC can be an important component of programs to reduce cesarean delivery rates in patients with term singleton fetuses with vertex presentations.
- Most women who have had one previous cesarean delivery with a low-transverse incision are candidates for VBAC.

- The ultimate decision as to whether to attempt a trial of labor or undergo an elective repeat cesarean delivery should be made by the patient and her physician after thorough counseling regarding the risks and benefits.
- Local opinion leaders who educate obstetric practitioners about VBAC can affect the proportion of women undergoing trial of labor.
- Using physician leadership in collaboration with nursing leadership to educate clinicians about VBAC may be most effective in regions with the highest cesarean delivery rates.

STRATEGIES

- Case-mix adjusted VBAC rates should be used for women with one prior low-transverse cesarean delivery at 37 weeks of gestation or more and with singleton fetuses with vertex presentations. These case-mix adjusted rates should be compared with the VBAC rate goals established by the DHHS expert working group to assess cesarean delivery rates for practitioners, hospitals, and regions. Recognizing marked variation in the route of delivery provides an indicator of current practice and an opportunity for improving future practice.
- Obstetric practitioners should identify women who are candidates for VBAC, counsel them regarding its risks and benefits, and offer them a trial of labor.

- Each hospital should develop a protocol for managing patients who attempt to deliver vaginally after a previous cesarean birth.

- Physician leadership, in collaboration with nursing leadership, should educate patients, fellow physicians, and nursing leadership about the risks and benefits of VBAC.

■ RECOMMENDATIONS

- Hospitals should monitor maternal and neonatal outcomes of women who undergo VBAC.

- The obstetric community needs to collect data on women with a previous uterine incision who attempt VBAC and women who successfully deliver vaginally after a previous cesarean delivery.

- The obstetric community needs to evaluate the trial of labor rate by using the formula for the VBAC rate.

- The obstetric community should use standardized definitions that will provide information necessary to evaluate reasons for increases or decreases in cesarean delivery rates in order to monitor trends. The denominator of the repeat cesarean delivery rate should be the number of women at risk (women delivering after prior cesarean delivery) to ensure that changes in the primary cesarean delivery rate do not obscure changes in the use of VBAC.

- Research should be conducted to identify antepartum and intrapartum factors that may predict success or failure of trial of labor, as well as risk of uterine rupture, in women with a prior cesarean delivery.

How Does the Management of Dystocia and Labor Abnormalities Affect the Cesarean Delivery Rate?

Dystocia

Dystocia is defined as difficult labor or childbirth. It can result from abnormalities primarily involving the cervix and uterus, the fetus, the maternal pelvis, or a combination of these factors. Functional dystocia, or dysfunctional labor, is a term used to describe conditions in which uterine contractions are inefficient. The latter is considered by some to be the most common complication of labor in nulliparous women. In fact, dystocia is the most common indication for cesarean delivery in the nulliparous patient, accounting for as much as 50% of the cesarean deliveries performed within this population. In contrast, dystocia accounts for less than 5% of cesarean deliveries performed on multiparous women, an example of the fundamental difference between a first and all subsequent births. Nearly all births diagnosed with cephalopelvic disproportion (96.5%) are cesarean deliveries (144).

Central to the management of presumed dystocia is augmentation of labor when uterine contractions do not result in effacement and dilatation of the cervix. The cervicographic illustration of cervical dilatation plotted against time has led to the recognition that the first stage of labor is made up of two components, the latent phase and the active phase. Although the onset of the latent phase of labor is often difficult to define precisely, based on a study of about 600 cases in 1955 (150 of which were excluded from analysis), a prolonged latent phase is considered to be one that exceeds 20 hours in the nulliparous patient. It is important to distinguish this aspect of normal labor to avoid a premature diagnosis of dystocia or failure to progress. "Failure to progress" is also an imprecise term and has been used to include lack of progressive cervical dilatation or lack of descent of the fetal head, or both. Often, the diagnosis of failure to progress is made before the active phase of labor has begun and before an adequate trial of labor has been achieved. Cesarean deliveries for dystocia should not be performed in the latent phase of labor. The active phase of the first stage of labor generally occurs when the cervix reaches 3–4 cm of dilatation. The Friedman curve may not be as applicable today as it was once thought to be.

The second stage of labor usually is brief for parous women, but longer for nulliparous women. Experience has shown that the duration of the second stage of labor should not be fixed by time, because it is not directly related to perinatal outcome when the fetal heart rate is reassuring and progress in descent is occurring (145).

■ STRATEGIES

- Institutions with high rates of cesarean delivery performed for dystocia when cervical dilatation was less than 3–4 cm should review their cesarean delivery rates for appropriateness.

- Clinicians and institutions should set appropriate criteria for cesarean delivery in the latent phase, active phase, and second stages of labor.

- Institutions and practitioners with high case-mix adjusted cesarean delivery rates for nulliparous women with term singleton fetuses with vertex presentations should be reviewed to see how many of these cesarean deliveries were performed when cervical dilatation was less than 4 cm.

- Institutions and practitioners with high case-mix adjusted cesarean delivery rates for nulliparous women with term singleton fetuses with vertex presentations should be reviewed to determine how many of these cesarean deliveries were performed without rupture of the membranes or without appropriate use of oxytocin.

Active Management

Labor augmentation techniques include amniotomy and oxytocin. Active management of labor is a method of labor management for nulliparous women consisting of four main components:

1. Standardized criteria for the diagnosis of labor (painful uterine contractions accompanied by bloody show, rupture of the membranes, or full cervical effacement)

2. Standardized methods of labor management, including early rupture of the membranes and careful monitoring of progress with an aggressive oxytocin regimen in the absence of expected progress

3. One-to-one nursing care throughout the course of labor

4. Prenatal education to teach women about the protocol

Although active management of labor has received considerable attention as a labor management technique, opinions vary as to its actual benefits. At the National Maternity Hospital in Dublin, Ireland, where active management of labor was first implemented, its use has been associated with a low rate of cesarean birth (146). The rate of cesarean delivery for dystocia was found to be particularly low, with only 1.5% of nulliparous women requiring a cesarean birth for that indication.

Most studies examining the effect of active management have compared cesarean delivery rates before and after active management of labor was introduced as routine procedure in a particular hospital. One such study reported that the overall cesarean delivery rate in nulliparous women decreased from 13.9% the year before active management was introduced to 10.8% the year that it was implemented (147). In addition, this study also found that the rate for dystocia among nulliparous women decreased from 4.9% to 1.8%. Another study found a lower cesarean birth rate among 552 nulliparous women treated with the active management of labor protocol (4.3% cesarean delivery rate) compared with a similar number of historical controls (13.0% cesarean delivery rate) (148). Other investigators reported on a population of 1,843 nulliparous women whose labor was actively managed and 2,057 historical controls. In their study, the overall cesarean delivery rate dropped from 24.3% to 18.8% after active management was introduced, and the cesarean rate for dystocia dropped from 13.9% to 8.8% (149).

Two large randomized studies also investigated the effects of implementing a protocol of active management. In the first trial, a group of 705 women were randomized to be treated under a protocol of either active management of labor or usual care. Not all aspects of the active management of labor protocol were implemented. Because women were randomized after the diagnosis of labor, there was no prenatal education component, and the criteria for the diagnosis of labor were the same for both groups. In addition, women in the active management group were not provided with one-to-one nursing care. Their cesarean delivery rate was 10.5%, somewhat lower than the rate of 14.1% in the control group. Although the crude difference was not statistically significant, the authors reported that the association did become significant after controlling for a large number of variables in a logistic regression analysis. In this study, women in both groups were treated by the same practitioners in the same labor and delivery unit, which may have influenced the results (150).

In the second trial, 1,934 low-risk women were randomized during pregnancy to be treated either with active management of labor or with usual care. The active management protocol included special childbirth classes for women. In addition, this protocol was implemented in a labor and birth unit remote from the hospital labor and birth suite, and the labor of women in the active management group were diagnosed and managed by certified nurse–midwives who worked exclusively for the study. Women laboring in the active management labor unit also received one-to-one nursing care during their entire course of labor (75).

Only women whose pregnancies reached term without complications and who had a spontaneous onset of labor with fetuses in the vertex position were eligible to receive the active management protocol. Because randomization occurred during the second trimester of pregnancy, a number of women in both groups did not meet these criteria. A secondary analysis that included only the subgroup of protocol-eligible women revealed no difference in the cesarean birth rate (10.9% for the active management group and 11.5% for the usual care group).

One interesting aspect of the difference in the cesarean delivery rates in the study at Brigham and Women's Hospital and the National Maternity Hospital relates to the timing of cesarean delivery. In the first study, the cesarean delivery rate during the first stage of labor for the active management group was 5.2%, similar to the 4.8% rate during the same stage of labor in the second study. In contrast, almost no cesarean deliveries were performed during the second stage of labor (second stage cesarean delivery rate = 0.2%) in the National Maternity Hospital study, whereas in the Boston study approximately half of the cesarean deliveries performed were done during the second stage (second stage cesarean delivery rate = 5.8%) (75, 146).

Although active management of labor has been used as an effective strategy to reduce high cesarean delivery rates in nulliparous women with dystocia, opinions regarding its efficacy vary. Efforts to identify abnormal labor and correct abnormal contraction patterns may help eliminate many cesarean deliveries without compromising outcome.

■ CONCLUSION

- In some institutions with high cesarean delivery rates for dystocia, active management of labor has been shown to be beneficial in reducing cesarean delivery rates.

■ STRATEGY

- Institutions with high case-mix adjusted cesarean delivery rates in nulliparous women with dystocia should explore the advantages of active management of labor.

How Does the Use of Epidural Analgesia Affect the Cesarean Delivery Rate?

The question of whether the use of epidural analgesia is associated with an increased risk of cesarean delivery remains controversial. The interpretation of many studies is limited by design problems, such as the inclusion of both nulliparous and multiparous women and the combination of women with spontaneous and induced labor. Because baseline cesarean delivery rates differ substantially among these populations, the effects of epidural analgesia may differ as well. A recurrent design problem is the failure to adequately account for the fact that women with difficult labor, who are more likely to have dystocia and require a cesarean birth, might also be more likely to request epidural analgesia.

Two observational studies examined the association between epidural analgesia and cesarean delivery. In an early study, the investigators examined 711 consecutive nulliparous patients with singleton fetuses with cephalic presentations; 63% of these women received epidural analgesia. The rate of cesarean delivery for dystocia was 3.8% in the nonepidural group and 9.1% in the epidural group. These differences remained statistically significant even when controlling for a variety of factors, including cervical dilatation on admission, infant birth weight and gestational age, maternal age, length of labor, and oxytocin use (151). The second study of 500 nulliparous women attempted specifically to address the issue of differences in labor characteristics between women choosing and not choosing epidural analgesia. Women were stratified according to both their rate of cervical dilatation during early labor (<1 cm/h or >1 cm/h for admission to 5 cm) and their epidural status (<5 cm, >5 cm, or none). After these factors were taken into account, the association between epidural analgesia and cesarean birth remained. There was a higher rate of cesarean delivery for dystocia among women receiving either early or late epidural anesthesia, regardless of whether cervical dilatation was slow or fast early in labor (151, 152).

Other investigators compared the association of epidural analgesia with cesarean delivery in a group of women treated with active management of labor (N = 346) to that of a group treated with usual care (N = 354). Epidural analgesia was used by 72% of the women in both groups. Both groups showed that the use of epidural analgesia was associated with more than a 4.5-fold increase in the risk of cesarean birth. This finding remained significant when controlling for a number of potentially confounding factors (153).

In contrast, increases in the use of epidural analgesia within an institution have not necessarily been accompanied by an increase in the rate of cesarean delivery. One study found no difference in the cesarean delivery rates between two different periods (16.7% from 1986 to 1987 and 16.0% from 1989 to 1990), despite the change from unavailability to on-demand administration of epidural analgesia (154). At the National Maternity Hospital, the use of epidural analgesia in nulliparous patients increased from 8% in 1987 to 50% in 1992, but the cesarean birth rate among that group increased only from 7.8% to 10.1% (146). This modest increase could in fact be related to the increased use of epidural analgesia. Historical comparisons must be interpreted with caution, however, taking into account that multiple changes may have occurred over time.

A retrospective study examined the association of epidural use with cesarean delivery in 1,733 low-risk nulliparous women with spontaneous labor and term singleton fetuses with cephalic presentations. The authors reported a cesarean delivery rate of 4% among women who did not receive epidural analgesia, compared with a rate of 17% among women who did. Women who received epidural analgesia tended to have a longer gestation and larger babies. They also tended to be admitted earlier in labor (less cervical dilatation and with a higher station of fetal head), and to dilate more slowly at admission than women who did not go on to receive epidural analgesia. To adjust for these differences in characteristics, the authors used the propensity score method. The propensity score was the probability that a woman would receive an epidural given her demographic, pregnancy, and baseline labor characteristics. The goal of the propensity score method is to simulate randomization as closely as possible by creating subgroups of individuals who display similar baseline characteristics but who have a different epidural status. Each woman was assigned a score (generated by multiple logistic regression) that took into account her race, prepregnancy weight and height, the birth weight and gestational age of her infant, her centimeters of dilatation at admission, her initial rate of cervical dilatation, the station of the fetal head at admission, and her treatment with the active management of labor protocol (155). These propensity scores were ordered from largest (most likely to receive an epidural) to smallest (least likely to receive an epidural). The authors found that regardless of propensity score, women receiving an epidural had a higher rate of cesarean birth. In a multivariate analysis controlling all the factors, women receiving an epidural were 3.7 times likelier to have a cesarean delivery (95%, CI = 2.4, 5.7).

Three randomized clinical trials have further examined the issue of epidural use. In a trial of 111 women, one study found a cesarean delivery rate of 17% in the epidural group compared with an 11% rate in the group receiving parenteral pain relief only (RR = 1.6, 95% CI = 0.6, 3.8) (156). Although the results were not statistically different, there was a somewhat high cesarean rate in the epidural group, despite the fact that the epidural was allowed to wear off after cervical dilatation reached 8 cm. In another study of 93 nulliparous women with a spontaneous onset of labor, the authors reported a 25% cesarean delivery rate with epidural analgesia and a 2.2% rate without epidural analgesia (RR = 11.4, 95% CI = 5.8, 16.9) (157). Although this study provides valuable information, it is not conclusive because of the small number of patients randomized and the fact that only 13 women in the study required a cesarean birth. Recently, in a larger trial (N = 1,330) that enrolled nulliparous and multiparous women in approximately equal numbers, the authors reported a 2.3-fold increase (9% versus 4%) in the rate of cesarean delivery associated with epidural use (158). However, because of an unanticipated high level of crossover, the primary analysis for cesarean delivery included only two thirds of women within each group who accepted the treatment assigned. It is important to note that acceptance of treatment varied by parity, a major risk factor for failure to progress (nulliparous women were more likely to accept epidural analgesia and less likely to accept parenteral pain relief).

A more recent study conducted a randomized trial of epidural analgesia use versus patient-controlled meperidine analgesia use during labor. In one group of 358 women randomized to receive epidural analgesia, 243 (68%) complied with the epidural protocol. In a second group of 337 women randomized to receive patient-controlled intravenous meperidine, 239 (73%) complied. There was no difference in the rates of cesarean birth between the two analgesic groups: 4% among the epidural group (95% CI, 1.9–6.2%) and 5% among the patient-controlled intravenous anesthesia group (95% CI, 2.6–7.2%). The cesarean delivery rates in both groups are strikingly low, even though both multiparous and nulliparous patients were included. The low rates raise the question of the generalizability of these observations to other populations (159).

The effect of the timing of epidural administration on cesarean delivery rates is another aspect of epidural use that has received attention. Two observational studies have found a 50% increase in risk of cesarean delivery among women who received an epidural when cervical dilatation was less than 5 cm compared with women who received an epidural later (155, 157). A randomized trial comparing combined spinal–epidural analgesia to epidural analgesia found that administration when cervical dilatation was less than 4 cm was associated with a higher cesarean delivery rate in both study groups (OR = 2.2, 95% CI, 1.4, 3.4) (160).

Another study in which the investigators conducted a randomized trial of 334 nulliparous women found no difference in the cesarean delivery rate for early epidural administration compared with late epidural administration (10% for early administration of epidural versus 8% for late administration of epidural) (161). However, in that study, only a small difference in the timing of epidural administration was found between the early and late groups (median of 4 cm cervical dilatation for early administration versus 5 cm cervical dilatation for late administration). It is similarly difficult to accurately evaluate the effect of timing of epidural administration in the randomized study mentioned previously given that only 13 patients received an epidural after their cervical dilatation reached 5 cm (160).

An alternative form of intrapartum analgesia is the combination of spinal and epidural analgesia. This method combines a single intrathecal injection of a lipid-soluble opioid with an epidural infusion of a solution containing both a local anesthetic and a narcotic. With respect to the controversy regarding the association between the use of conventional lumbar epidural analgesia for pain relief during labor and the diagnosis of dystocia, the combined spinal–epidural analgesia has been offered as a solution.

However, in a recent randomized controlled trial of 761 nulliparous women, researchers were unable to demonstrate a reduction in the cesarean delivery rate when conventional epidural analgesia was received compared with when combined epidural analgesia was received. The incidence of dystocia necessitating cesarean delivery among those who received combined spinal–epidural analgesia did not differ from the rate among those who received conventional epidural analgesia (160).

The effect of epidural analgesia on the risk of cesarean delivery remains controversial. A majority of the few randomized trials comparing cesarean birth rates with and without epidural use have all found a positive association. However, because most studies are not randomized, it has been suggested that the positive associations reported are a result of uncontrolled confounding.

There is considerable evidence suggesting that there is in fact an association between the use of epidural analgesia for pain relief during labor and the risk of cesarean delivery. Because it is recognized that epidural analgesia is the most effective form of pain relief for labor, there is no desire to limit its use by women in labor. However, it has been observed that the risk for cesarean delivery is lowered if epidural analgesia is administered after the active phase of labor has been entered and fetal head station has progressed into the lower half of the pelvis. This observation should be kept in mind when considering the timing for the epidural and the risk–benefit ratio for the individual patient (162).

■ STRATEGIES

- When feasible, obstetric practitioners should delay the administration of epidural anesthesia in nulliparous women until the cervical dilatation reaches at least 4–5 cm.

- Practitioners should recommend using other forms of analgesia instead of an epidural prior to cervical dilatation of 4–5 cm.

- Institutions and practitioners with high case-mix adjusted rates of cesarean deliveries in nulliparous women with term singleton fetuses with vertex presentations should be reviewed to determine how many of these patients received an epidural when cervical dilatation was less than 4 cm.

Does Electronic Fetal Monitoring Affect the Cesarean Delivery Rate?

Perhaps by coincidence, the increase in the use of EFM in the early 1970s paralleled the increase in the cesarean delivery rate in the United States. The early reports on EFM using historical controls, even when comparing high-risk monitored patients to low-risk unmonitored patients, suggested better outcomes with EFM (163, 164). It was not until prospective randomized controlled trials of EFM versus intermittent auscultation were conducted in more than 18,000 patients that the benefits of using EFM even came into question. The results of these randomized controlled trials made it evident that both immediate and long-term outcomes were not improved with EFM. In fact, studies showed that the significant increase in the cesarean birth rate associated with EFM over intermittent auscultation was attributed to nonreassuring fetal status in some populations and to dystocia in others (165–173).

Normal EFM patterns rarely result in fetuses with low Apgar scores or fetal acidosis. Nonreassuring patterns also correlate poorly with low Apgar scores and fetal acidosis, but it is rare that a hypoxic–acidemic fetus would not have a concurrent nonreassuring fetal heart rate (FHR) pattern (174–175).

Some studies show that additionally requiring fetal scalp blood pH monitoring to validate nonreassuring EFM patterns decreases the likely cesarean delivery rate (168). Other studies indicate that using amnioinfusion for patients with variable decelerations, thick meconium, or oligohydramnios also may decrease the cesarean delivery rate in electronically monitored patients (176–178).

In response to the results of the randomized controlled trials, ACOG concluded that intermittent auscultation at least every 15 minutes in the first stage of labor and at least every 5 minutes in the second stage of labor was an acceptable alternative to continuous EFM in high-risk patients (179). In low-risk patients, auscultation at least every 30 minutes in the first stage of labor and at least every 15 minutes in the second stage of labor in lieu of EFM was considered an appropriate alternative (179). In order to detect the patient with decreased variability on admission, which might reflect a preexisting abnormality of the central nervous system, many obstetricians advocate running a 30-minute EFM strip before beginning intermittent auscultation. Despite these findings, continuous EFM continues to be highly utilized because of, among other reasons, the perception that it reduces personnel requirements during labor and birth.

The exact reasons for the increased cesarean delivery rate related to EFM in some populations are not completely understood, but may include the following:

1. An inconsistent definition and interpretation of EFM patterns

2. The additive effect of mild EFM changes in patients with other developing problems, such as failed progress, meconium staining, suspected macrosomia, or maternal medical disease

3. Nonreassuring EFM patterns in patients with preexisting nonhypoxic fetal abnormalities

4. The decreased likelihood for electronically monitored patients to ambulate in labor

5. Overreaction of frequently observed patterns of variable deceleration in the second stage of labor; these do not necessarily mandate intervention

The following periodic FHR patterns are considered to be indications for expeditious delivery:

1. Persistent, uncorrectable late decelerations

2. Persistent, uncorrectable, severe variable decelerations

Patients may continue to labor with the above two patterns if a fetal scalp blood pH is normal (180) or if spontaneous or evoked FHR accelerations are present (181). If there is an associated absent baseline FHR variability or an uncorrectable prolonged deceleration, expeditious birth is indicated. It is estimated that the usual cesarean delivery rate for nonreassuring fetal status is in the range of 1–3% of deliveries.

■ CONCLUSIONS

- Using fetal scalp blood sampling or fetal scalp stimulation for evoked FHR accelerations when EFM patterns are nonreassuring has been linked to reduced need for cesarean delivery.
- Intermittent auscultation rather than continuous EFM has been associated with a decrease in cesarean delivery rates.

■ STRATEGIES

- Obstetric practitioners may use fetal scalp blood sampling or fetal scalp stimulation for evoked FHR accelerations to avoid intervention when EFM patterns are nonreassuring.
- Obstetric practitioners should reassess fetal status following intrauterine resuscitation with position change, tocolysis, increase in the intravenous infusion of fluids, decrease or discontinuation of oxytocin, or amnioinfusion for persistent variable decelerations remote from delivery.
- Obstetric practitioners may use intermittent auscultation rather than continuous EFM.
- Institutions should conduct chart reviews and individual clinician feedback on patients having cesarean deliveries for abnormal heart rate patterns.

What Is the Impact of Suspected Macrosomia in the Nondiabetic Pregnant Woman on Cesarean Delivery Rates?

This section does not address macrosomia in diabetic pregnant women because concerns about the risk of shoulder dystocia are higher. Shoulder dystocia and other birth trauma associated with the delivery of macrosomic infants are linked to a higher rate of cesarean deliveries. However, the prenatal diagnosis of macrosomia is extremely imprecise (182). This is further compounded by the misperception that delivering an apparently macrosomic infant by inducing labor before it reaches full-term growth is an effective way to reduce delivery problems.

One study has found a statistically significant effect on both the diagnosis of labor abnormalities and the incidence of elective cesarean deliveries in women who received an incorrect ultrasonographic diagnosis of fetal macrosomia, when in fact the fetus was appropriate for gestational age (183). Another study has reported similar findings (184). When fetal macrosomia was predicted before delivery, the cesarean birth rate was 52%, compared with 30% when macrosomia was present but not predicted. All infants in this study weighed 4,200 g at birth or more. The increased cesarean delivery rate was accounted for by an increased incidence of labor induction and a greater proportion of failed inductions. These investigators concluded that an antenatal prediction of fetal macrosomia was associated with a marked increase in cesarean deliveries without a significant reduction in the incidence of shoulder dystocia or fetal injury.

One study evaluated the ability of late third-trimester ultrasound examinations to diagnose the large-for-gestational-age (LGA) fetus, or fetal macrosomia, defined as greater than or equal to the 90th percentile (183). The ultrasonographic prediction of fetal macrosomia had a sensitivity of 50%, a specificity of 90%, and a positive predictive value of only 52%. Another study examined 242 nondiabetic women with ultrasonographically estimated fetal weights (EFWs) greater than or equal to 4,000 g, or greater than or equal to the 90th percentile (185). Among those delivering within 3 days of the ultrasound examination, 77% had an EFW that exceeded the actual birth weight. Only 48% had an actual weight within the corresponding 500 g increment that was predicted. Other investigators reported that single- or multiple-growth ultrasound examinations provided birth weight percentile estimates within 10% of the actual birth weight percentile only approximately 50% of the time (187). Other observations have further noted that increased body fat in infants of diabetic mothers was associated with an ultrasonographic overestimation of fetal weight (187).

A retrospective case review compared perinatal outcomes in macrosomic nondiabetic fetuses whose labor had been spontaneous or induced (188). All infants weighed 4,000 g or more. Although frequencies of shoulder dystocia, 1-minute Apgar scores less than 7, and abnormal umbilical cord blood gas determinations were not different between the two groups, the cesarean delivery rate was significantly higher (23.9% when labor was induced and 10% when spontaneous labor was awaited). Another retrospective analysis matched nondiabetic patients who underwent labor induction for fetal macrosomia to the next nondiabetic patient delivering a child of equal or greater birth weight who entered labor spontaneously (189). There were no differences between the induction and spontaneous labor groups in maternal age, gestational age, rate of nulliparity, incidence of shoulder dystocia, Apgar scores, or VBAC. The cesarean delivery rate was significantly higher in the induction group than in the spontaneous labor group (36% versus 17%), despite a statistically significant lower birth weight in the induction group. The authors suggest using a plan of expectant management when fetal macrosomia is suspected.

Other studies (190, 191) have reported similar increases in operative vaginal delivery when elective induction with oxytocin, amniotomy, or both are used to manage labor in cases of suspected macrosomia, with no impact on the occurrence of shoulder dystocia. When logistic regression was used to control for birth weight, parity, and practitioner, elective induction was associated with a higher risk of cesarean birth than was spontaneous labor, with an adjusted odds ratio of 2.7 and a confidence interval of 1.2 to 5.9. The only published prospective randomized study of induction of labor for suspected macrosomia at term used EFW of 4,000–4,500 g (192). Induction of labor was used with 139 patients and expectant management with 134 patients. Labor induction had no effect on either decreasing the rate of cesarean delivery or reducing neonatal morbidity. The authors concluded that an ultrasonographic estimation of a fetal weight between 4,000 and 4,500 g should not be considered an indication for induction of labor.

■ CONCLUSION

- Induction of labor for suspected macrosomia does not improve outcome, expends considerable resources, and may increase the cesarean delivery rate.

■ STRATEGIES

- Institutions and practitioners with high case-mix adjusted rates of cesarean deliveries for nulliparous nondiabetic women with term singleton fetuses with vertex presentations should be reviewed to see how many of these patients underwent elective cesarean delivery or failed induction of labor leading to subsequent cesarean delivery for suspected macrosomia.

- Institutions should encourage trial of labor by nondiabetic women regardless of estimated fetal weight in cases of suspected macrosomia with adequate labor progress and a reassuring fetal heart rate.

- The peripartum diagnosis of macrosomia often is imprecise; obstetric practitioners should not induce labor for suspected macrosomia or perform cesarean delivery for the sole indication of estimated fetal weight.

How Does Induction of Labor Affect the Cesarean Delivery Rate?

The induction of labor prior to 41 weeks of gestation is associated with increased cesarean delivery rates. Current ACOG policy states that, "the benefits of labor induction must be weighed against the potential maternal or fetal risks associated with this procedure" (193).

Using the Swedish Medical Birth Registry, researchers reported a statistically significant difference in the stillbirth rate from a gestational age of 41 weeks in nulliparous women, whereas for multiparous women the risk did not occur until 42 completed weeks of gestation (194). The odds ratio for a nulliparous woman to have an intrauterine death increased to 1.50 at 41 weeks of gestation and 1.79 at 42 weeks of gestation, compared with a risk of 1.0 at 40 weeks of gestation. In most studies of postterm pregnancies, women are recruited and monitoring begins prior to 42 completed weeks of gestation, despite no demonstrable evidence that any form of antenatal testing is beneficial for patients between 40 and 42 completed weeks of gestation (195).

One author compared labor induction and expectant management in women who had reached 41 6/7 weeks of gestation. Birth before 42 weeks of gestation occurred in 86% of the induced group and in 64% of those managed expectantly. The cesarean delivery rates were statistically significantly different according to management schemes: 21.2% in the induction group and 24.5% in the expectant management with serial antenatal testing group (196). Moreover, the most cost-effective management was with planned induction of labor beyond 41 weeks of gestation (197). In a similar group of patients managed in the Maternal Fetal Medicine Network, no significant statistical difference was shown between induction of labor and expectant management (198). Because adverse perinatal outcome in the otherwise uncomplicated pregnancies of 41–42 weeks of gestation was low with either management scheme, both were felt to be equally acceptable.

■ STRATEGIES

- Obstetric practitioners should not induce labor in patients with unfavorable cervices before 41 completed weeks of gestation unless maternal or fetal complications that constitute an indication for induction are present.

- If the cervix is unfavorable, obstetric practitioners should consider induction of labor for women who have completed 41–42 weeks of gestation.

- Obstetric practitioners should inform women at 41–42 completed weeks of gestation in an otherwise uncomplicated pregnancy of the benefits and risks associated with induction of labor and expectant management and respect their preferences.

- Institutions and practitioners with high case-mix adjusted rates of cesarean deliveries for nulliparous women with term singleton fetuses with vertex presentations should be reviewed to see how many of these patients underwent elective induction of labor prior to 41 completed weeks of gestation.

How Does the Management of Breech Presentation Affect the Cesarean Delivery Rate?

Approximately 3.5% of pregnancies present at term with fetuses in the breech presentation. Planned breech delivery versus cesarean delivery for breech presentation continues to be controversial, and the practitioner must consider each case on its own merits. Because the data on selective trial of labor with fetuses with breech presentations are inconsistent (199, 200), this report only discusses external cephalic version (ECV) as a means to manage term fetuses with breech presentations.

External Cephalic Version

Reduction of the cesarean delivery rate associated with breech presentation at term is most likely to be affected by ECV at 37 weeks of gestation. Spontaneous version to the vertex presentation after 37 weeks of gestation occurs only 15–20% of the time. Conversion of the fetus from the breech presentation to the cephalic presentation eliminates the concern for head entrapment in an incompletely dilated cervix, as well as the concern for nuchal and extended arms. This procedure offers the potential to reduce the prevalence of breech presentation at term by approximately 50–60%. Success rates for ECV are generally in the range of 50–75%, with a reversion back to the breech presentation occurring approximately 2% of the time (201–203).

The immediate benefit of a successful ECV at 37 weeks of gestation is an increased probability that the fetus will be in a vertex presentation for labor and delivery. Studies show that there are fewer cesarean deliveries among women who have undergone successful ECV compared with women who have not undergone attempted version (200, 204–212). External cephalic version can be performed with minimal risk to the mother and fetus (213).

Fetal heart rate changes are not uncommon during an attempted ECV, but usually stabilize when the procedure is discontinued (204, 206, 214–216). Serious adverse effects do not occur often, but there have been a few reported cases of placental abruption and preterm labor. Fetal assessment before and after the procedure is recommended (213).

■ CONCLUSIONS

- Controversy remains regarding the choice of mode of delivery for fetuses with breech presentations.

- External cephalic version of the term fetus with breech presentation may significantly reduce the rate of cesarean deliveries for breech presentation.

■ STRATEGIES

- Obstetric practitioners should encourage all women with fetuses with persistent breech presentation at 37 weeks of gestation or greater to undergo ECV, if there are no contraindications.

- Institutions and practitioners with high cesarean delivery rates for term fetuses with breech presentations should be reviewed to determine how many underwent attempted ECV.

- Institutions should consider making the assistance of obstetricians experienced in ECV available to obstetric practitioners desiring their expertise.

- Institutions should monitor their cesarean delivery rate for term fetuses with breech presentations, and should consider whether increased use of ECV would improve this rate.

■ RECOMMENDATION

- Further research is recommended to determine the safety and efficacy of increased use of ECV in larger patient populations.

What Are the Effects of Preterm Delivery on the Cesarean Delivery Rate?

Preterm birth increases the risk of nonvertex presentation as well as the fragility of the infant, thus increasing its susceptibility to trauma. The survival rate of very premature infants has increased in recent years, coincident with changes in the neonatal management of the very small infant, such as artificial surfactant, innovations in ventilatory management, and improved understanding of neonatal fluid and temperature homeostasis (217). Although some studies have shown a decreased incidence of intraventricular hemorrhage associated with cesarean delivery performed for a variety of indications (218), others have not, including studies of pregnancies complicated by preeclampsia or eclampsia (219) and pregnancies complicated by frank or complete breech presentation (220). The comparative study of patients with preeclampsia or eclampsia actually showed a significant reduction in the risk of respiratory distress syndrome in newborns who experienced labor (219). Balancing any potential improvement in neonatal outcome associated with cesarean delivery is the increased risk of maternal morbidity and mortality. Cesarean delivery at the limits of viability may jeopardize the mother's health, fertility, and life without providing any benefit to her child. The concern for the mother is intensified because of the increased need for a classical cesarean incision in premature cesarean delivery, which further increases the risk of long-term maternal morbidity (221).

At the margin of viability, intervention by cesarean delivery for obstetric indications (eg, breech presentation, prolapsed cord, fetal intolerance of labor, placental abruption) may improve survival (222). However, intervention based on low birth weight (LBW) alone has not been proven to be beneficial. When fetuses younger than 26 weeks of gestation or less than 800 g were evaluated separately, however, the willingness to intervene was associated with an increased risk of survival with significant morbidity. In response to concerns such as these, the Canadian Paediatric Society and the Society of Obstetricians and Gynaecologists of Canada have advocated several different interventions depending on gestational age (223): 1) no intervention at 22 weeks of gestation; 2) significant discussion with the family prior to intervention on behalf of the fetus at 23–24 weeks of gestation; and 3) intervention on behalf of the fetus at 25–26 weeks or more of gestation.

As the literature illustrates, clinical trials and even a meta-analysis of the available trials of cesarean versus vaginal delivery for the very-low-birth-weight (VLBW) fetus have been small and inconclusive (224, 225). It is therefore difficult at this time to form any firm conclusions regarding outcome.

■ CONCLUSION

- There is no evidence to support cesarean delivery of the preterm fetus on the basis of gestational age alone, although cesarean delivery on behalf of the VLBW fetus in the presence of an obstetric indication may be beneficial.

■ STRATEGY

- The route of delivery of VLBW fetuses should be individualized. Cesarean delivery should be considered only in the presence of an obstetric indication.

■ RECOMMENDATION

- Further study of the optimal mode of delivery of the VLBW fetus is necessary.

Can the Intrapartum Management of Multifetal Gestations Affect the Cesarean Delivery Rate?

Data from NCHS indicate that in 1997, live-born twins accounted for only 2.7% of total live-born infants but had a 53.9% cesarean delivery rate. The number of multifetal pregnancies in the United States is growing, due in large part to the increased use of assisted reproductive technologies. Attempts are being made to monitor and evaluate recommendations to limit the number of embryos being implanted per attempt. Strict laws in the United Kingdom allow no more than three embryos to be transferred during one cycle; the American Society for Reproductive Medicine recommends transferring no more than 3–5 embryos per cycle, depending on the mother's prognosis (226). Studies of in vitro fertilization, gamete intrafallopian transfer, and zygote intrafallopian transfer report that the overall rate of multiple pregnancies averages between 15% and 34% (50). The rate of triplet and higher-order births varies between 3% and 9%. There are also indications of a connection between the increased age of mothers and increased twinning rates (50). Multifetal pregnancy is associated with a much higher rate of cesarean births than singleton pregnancy. Data from NCHS indicates that in 1996, the U.S. cesarean birth rate for twins was 53.4%; 90.3% of triplet and higher-order gestations were delivered by cesarean. This report will be limited to a discussion of twins, because of the lack of data to evaluate cesarean delivery in higher-order multifetal pregnancies.

Factors contributing to the high cesarean delivery rate in twin pregnancies include an increase in preterm and growth-restricted fetuses, a higher rate of malpresentation, and an increased frequency of medical risks, such as preeclampsia and abruptio placenta. Unfortunately, population-based data describing the range of indications, including dystocia, for cesarean delivery of twins are not available. Most of the published studies pertain to presentation, of which practice varies considerably.

Presentation of twins is classified into three general groups: 1) twin A vertex, twin B vertex (43%); 2) twin A vertex, twin B nonvertex (38%); and 3) twin A nonvertex (19%). Although an estimated 70–80% of vertex–vertex twins may be safely delivered vaginally (227), the management of twins in the vertex–breech presentation or the vertex–transverse presentation remains in dispute. A number of cohort studies indicate that a trial of labor is safe for twins more than 1,500–2,000 g (228–230). The second twin can be delivered by breech extraction or external cephalic version (231). Other evidence suggests that a strategy of breech extraction without an attempt at external cephalic version is safe and is associated with a lower rate of cesarean birth for the second twin (232). However, there are insufficient data to advocate a specific route of delivery of the second twin whose birth weight is less than 1,500 g, even though several controlled studies suggest that breech extraction is safe regardless of birth weight (233, 234). There are also insufficient data to support the safety of vaginal delivery when the first twin is nonvertex, although some studies suggest that it is safe (231). External cephalic version of a nonvertex first twin has been reported (235), but cesarean delivery still appears to be preferable when the first twin is nonvertex.

Although the predominant clinical practice in the management of twin pregnancies has been cesarean delivery, primarily because of concern over the initial or eventual nonvertex presentation of the second twin, there is no evidence to validate this practice. Second twins delivered vaginally show similar risks of morbidity and mortality regardless of whether they are delivered with breech or vertex presentation (236).

■ CONCLUSION

- Despite the predominant practice of delivering twins by cesarean delivery, vaginal delivery of appropriately selected twin pregnancies may be considered.

■ STRATEGIES

- Institutions and practitioners should collect hospital- and practitioner-specific data on cesarean deliveries for the indication of twin gestation.

- Obstetric practitioners not comfortable with vaginal delivery of the second twin should consider referral to or co-management with an experienced obstetrician.

Alternatives to Cesarean Delivery

Is Operative Vaginal Delivery an Appropriate Alternative to Cesarean Delivery?

Forceps deliveries have been a central aspect of operative obstetrics for centuries (237, 238) and are thought by many experts, along with vacuum-assisted vaginal deliveries, to be an essential component of the future of obstetrics. Forceps and vacuum deliveries often enable a vaginal delivery in situations where the only alternative is a cesarean birth. Although forceps and vacuum delivery may be associated with fetal or maternal trauma, the incidence of significant morbidity is small when these devices are used appropriately, and there is no indication that operative vaginal delivery imposes sufficient risk to the fetus or mother to warrant the risk inherent in the alternative birth route of cesarean delivery (239).

In 1988, ACOG changed the classification of forceps deliveries to avoid the inclusion of both trivial and extremely difficult deliveries under the single category of midforceps (240). Before this reclassification, a rotational delivery from occiput posterior at 0 station was classified the same as a delivery from left occiput anterior with the head on the perineum. In a validation of ACOG's reclassification, investigators demonstrated that the lower the fetal head or the less rotation required, the less risk of injury to the mother and child (240–242).

Although there is an association between either forceps deliveries or vacuum deliveries and a number of poor outcomes for the mother and her infant, clinical trials have failed to document an increased risk of long-term morbidity relative to those of alternative delivery routes. One such trial of elective low-forceps deliveries versus vaginal deliveries showed no detrimental effect of the forceps on the fetus, and in fact suggested a slight improvement in the neonatal pH and a somewhat shortened second stage of labor (243). A study comparing failed operative vaginal delivery with subsequent cesarean delivery to cesarean delivery during the second stage of labor with no antecedent attempt at operative vaginal delivery also showed no difference in either short-term neonatal or maternal morbidity (244). In general, the risk of fetal injury would seem comparable between forceps deliveries and vacuum deliveries; however, the distribution of injury is different with a greater likelihood of facial marks and facial nerve palsy with forceps delivery, and of cephalohematoma with vacuum delivery (240, 245).

Still, fewer practicing obstetricians include obstetric forceps as part of their clinical equipment, in part because the vacuum often is substituted for forceps. Contemporaneous surveys show that the rate of operative vaginal delivery among a majority of both ACOG Fellows (246) and obstetric residents in the United States (247) is below 15%. Most Fellows no longer attempt operative vaginal delivery in the management of deep transverse arrest (246), and most training programs (residency or fellowship) no longer teach midpelvic forceps delivery, instead preferring vacuum delivery in this setting (242). It has been proposed that the same prerequisites and classification system be used for both forceps deliveries and vacuum deliveries to enhance safety (248).

Some authors have suggested that the decline in the operative vaginal delivery rate has been replaced, in whole or in part, by the noted increase in the cesarean delivery rate (248–250). Indeed, it is likely that the number of operative deliveries will remain constant. Rather, as the number of forceps deliveries and vacuum deliveries decreases, the number of cesarean deliveries will increase.

This trend toward a declining operative vaginal delivery rate might be reversed, however, with improved understanding of the conduct of normal labor, particularly in the second stage. As long as labor is progressing, and in the presence of reassuring FHR patterns, continuation of the second stage of labor should be permitted.

■ STRATEGIES

- Hospitals with a high cesarean delivery rate should consider introducing training during and after residency in the appropriate use of forceps and the vacuum in the management of second-stage arrest.

- Institutions may consider making the assistance of obstetricians experienced in operative vaginal deliveries available to obstetric practitioners desiring their expertise.

Evaluation Tools

Standardized and Case-Mix Adjusted Cesarean Delivery Rates

Cesarean delivery rates can be used to monitor trends nationally and regionally as well as to compare the performance of institutions and practitioners. Each institution must determine the appropriateness of its overall cesarean delivery rate and the rates of its obstetric practitioners. This data will be more useful if it includes whether this is a woman's first or subsequent pregnancy; if she has had a previous cesarean delivery; and for what indication (eg, suspected macrosomia, breech presentation) was the cesarean delivery performed. Ongoing monitoring of cesarean delivery rates for institutions and for individual practitioners is a necessary first step in evaluating cesarean delivery rates (251).

The most effective means of lowering cesarean delivery rates may differ from institution to institution. Institutions should regularly monitor management practices related to cesarean delivery, understand the reasons for elevated cesarean delivery rates, identify interventions that may be effective in a particular setting, and monitor changes in practice over time (142).

Cesarean delivery rates and data derived from these rates should also be used to assess and give feedback to individual practitioners. Any medical or nonmedical misperceptions about the appropriateness of cesarean versus vaginal delivery in a certain circumstance needs to be identified and corrected as soon as possible (142).

The types of data that will be useful in evaluating cesarean delivery rates are listed in Appendix B. Examples of key categories of deliveries to be monitored might include: induction of labor in nulliparous women as an elective procedure or for the indications of suspected macrosomia or postterm pregnancy at less than 41 completed weeks of gestation, cesarean deliveries performed when cervical dilatation is less than 4 cm, and the percentage of eligible women with a prior cesarean birth attempting a vaginal delivery.

Evaluation of cesarean delivery rates also often involves comparisons across institutions and practitioners. It is inappropriate to use unadjusted cesarean delivery rates to assess individual institutions or obstetric practitioners, because all practitioners have some patients in their practice who are at increased risk for cesarean delivery, regardless of management practices. Women at higher risk include those with a previous cesarean delivery through a classical uterine incision (as opposed to a low-transverse uterine incision), as well as women with certain medical or obstetric conditions. For unbiased comparisons to be performed, these differences must be taken into account.

One study evaluated the impact of adjustment of hospital cesarean delivery rates for women without a previous cesarean delivery, ranking the primary delivery cesarean rates for 21 hospitals in a single metropolitan area before and after adjustment for 39 clinical factors associated with cesarean delivery in a logistic regression analysis. The study found that this adjustment changed hospital rankings substantially and even altered which hospitals were significantly lower or higher than expected (252). Another study examined the effect of adjusting cesarean delivery rates for women with singleton births of at least 2,500 g. Complex logistic regression analyses of data from linked birth certificate and hospital discharge data found somewhat more modest changes in hospital-specific rates as a result of case-mix adjustment (253). Both studies conclude, however, that adjustment for case mix is needed when comparing cesarean delivery rates between hospitals.

Studies have examined how best to compare cesarean delivery rates between clinicians or institutions. One study suggests that only cesarean delivery rates for low-risk nulliparous women be compared for different hospitals (254). Another study suggests reporting practitioner-specific cesarean delivery rates minus cesarean deliveries for indications that are justifiable on the basis of current medical practice (44% of cesarean births in their study population). Justifiable indications included in that study were nonvertex–vertex twins, estimated fetal weight greater than or equal to 4,500 g, and abnormal fetal lie, as well as other relative maternal and fetal contraindications to labor. The authors also recommend separately reporting rates for nulliparous women and multiparous women (255).

A method of adjustment, which uses hospital discharge data to compare cesarean delivery rates between hospitals, has been advanced by the Maine Medical Assessment Foundation (<www.mmaf. org/cesarean.html>). Using discharge diagnosis codes, women were categorized into groups based on risk of cesarean delivery. Using the overall Maine cesarean delivery rate for each category as a benchmark, an expected cesarean delivery rate was calculated for each hospital and the institution's observed rates compared with the standard rate for that category.

Another study proposes a simple method for case-mix adjustment of cesarean birth rates; using this technique, standardized rates can be obtained for comparison purposes. This procedure is described in Appendix C. The calculation requires the answer to only eight yes or no questions (Appendix C), and, with a simple calculation, provides a case-mix adjusted cesarean delivery rate that can be compared among clinicians or among institutions.

The answers to the eight questions classify women into subgroups according to the risk of cesarean delivery. These categories are based on three parity categories (nulliparous women, multiparous women without previous cesarean delivery, and multiparous with previous cesarean delivery) and six obstetric condition groups (multiple pregnancy, breech presentation, preterm delivery, medical condition precluding a trial of labor, term singleton fetus with vertex presentation with medical complication, and term singleton fetus with vertex presentation without medical complication). A clinician's or institution's cesarean delivery rate for each of the subgroups is determined. The adjusted rate is then calculated using standardization, a simple biostatistical technique that permits calculation of cesarean delivery rates under the assumption that every provider or institution sees the same population of patients (a standard population). For this method, having a standard population translates into having the same proportion of patients in each parity or obstetric condition subgroup. The specific proportions chosen for each subgroup of the standard population is not critical, as long as they total 100%. As demonstrated in Appendix C, this calculation results in a single number, a standardized cesarean delivery rate. These standardized cesarean delivery rates can be compared with each other as long as the same standard population was used to derive them. Using this adjustment, two obstetricians with identical management practices will appear comparable in terms of cesarean delivery rate, regardless of the composition of their practice. The term "standardized" in this context refers to the rate derived from the case-mix adjustment technique.

It should be remembered that nulliparous women with term singleton fetuses with vertex presentations and multiparous women with one previous low-transverse cesarean delivery and term singleton fetuses with vertex presentations account for two thirds of all cesarean deliveries in the United States, and the most striking variations in cesarean delivery rates. The methodology developed by the Department of Health and Human Services expert working group, which included ACOG representatives, uses 1996 NCHS U.S. natality data for both of these groups (Tables 5, 6, and 7) to establish benchmarks and goals for cesarean deliveries. The availability of these benchmarks provides an excellent opportunity for institutions and practitioners to assess their cesarean delivery rates; ACOG recommends that obstetric institutions and practitioners, at a minimum, monitor their cesarean delivery rates for these two groups.

A number of clinical practices are associated with increased cesarean deliveries. Institutions and practitioners whose rates differ appreciably from these benchmarks for the two primary patient groups should consider reviewing their cesarean delivery rates. The following variables should be examined when cesarean deliveries are performed:

- when cervical dilatation was less than 4 cm
- in the presence of intact membranes

Table 5. National Rates and Benchmarks of Cesarean Deliveries in Nulliparous Women at 37 Weeks of Gestation or Greater with Singleton Fetuses with Vertex Presentations and Multiparous Women with One Prior Low-Transverse Cesarean Delivery at 37 Weeks of Gestation or Greater with Singleton Fetuses with Vertex Presentations, 1996

Nulliparous Women at 37 Weeks of Gestation or Greater with Singleton Fetuses with Vertex Presentations (National Rate)	25th Percentile (Expert Working Group Benchmark)	Multiparous Women with One Previous Low-Transverse Cesarean Delivery at 37 Weeks of Gestation or Greater with Singleton Fetuses with Vertex Presentations—VBAC* (National Rate)	75th Percentile (Expert Working Group Benchmark)
17.9	15.5	30.3	37.0

* Abbreviation: VBAC, vaginal birth after previous cesarean delivery

Table 6. Regional Rates of Cesarean Deliveries in Nulliparous Women at 37 Weeks of Gestation or Greater with Singleton Fetuses with Vertex Presentations and Multiparous Women with One Prior Low-Transverse Cesarean Delivery at 37 Weeks of Gestation or Greater with Singleton Fetuses with Vertex Presentations, 1996

Region	Nulliparous Women at 37 Weeks of Gestation or Greater with Singleton Fetuses with Vertex Presentations (Regional Rate)	Multiparous Women with One Previous Low-Transverse Cesarean Delivery at 37 Weeks of Gestation or Greater with Singleton Fetuses with Vertex Presentations—VBAC* (Regional Rate)
Northeast	18.8	35.4
Midwest	16.2	33.4
South	19.7	25.9
West	16.2	29.6

* Abbreviation: VBAC, vaginal birth after cesarean delivery.

- without appropriate use of oxytocin
- after the patient has received an epidural when cervical dilatation was less than 4 cm
- after the patient has undergone elective induction of labor at less than 41 completed weeks of gestation
- without trial of labor for suspected macrosomia in nondiabetic women
- for failed induction of labor for suspected macrosomia in nondiabetic women
- for the sole indication of twin gestation
- for the indication of term fetuses with breech presentations, without offering external cephalic version

This information should be made available to outlier practitioners and institutions, to enable them to review, and if appropriate, adjust their practices. Feedback regarding cesarean delivery rates has been shown to encourage obstetric practitioners to reconsider their practice patterns (256).

■ STRATEGIES

- Groups at high and low risk for cesarean delivery should be identified using a case-mix approach. The low-risk group can be evaluated for any wide variation.

- Institutions and practitioners should consider reviewing their cesarean delivery rates with these benchmarks for 1) nulliparous women with term singleton fetuses with vertex presentations and, 2) multiparous women with one previous low-transverse cesarean delivery and term singleton fetuses with vertex presentations.

- Institutions and practitioners whose cesarean delivery rates differ widely from these benchmarks should consider reviewing their cesarean delivery rates for variables described previously.

- Institutions and practitioners seeking greater insight into their cesarean delivery rates can use more sophisticated procedures, such as the case-mix adjusted approach (251), to evaluate their cesarean results.

- Obstetric practitioners and institutions should adjust their cesarean delivery rates for case mix to yield more valid comparisons of cesarean delivery rates between practitioners and across institutions.

- Each hospital and clinical practice should establish a benchmark cesarean delivery rate based on clinical factors specific to that hospital or practice.

- Clinician-specific factors should be reviewed if a high variation in cesarean delivery rates is identified.

■ RECOMMENDATIONS

- Obstetric practitioners and institutions should continuously collect data and monitor both their case-mix adjusted cesarean delivery rates and labor practices, which may influence cesarean delivery rates.

- Institutions and practitioners should make use of national, regional, and state benchmarks for cesarean deliveries.

Table 7. State Rates of Cesarean Deliveries in Nulliparous Women at 37 Weeks of Gestation or Greater with Singleton Fetuses with Vertex Presentations and Multiparous Women with One Prior Low-Transverse Cesarean Delivery at 37 Weeks of Gestation or Greater with Singleton Fetuses with Vertex Presentations, 1996

State	Nulliparous Women at 37 Weeks of Gestation or Greater with Singleton Fetuses with Vertex Presentations	Multiparous Women with One Previous Low-Transverse Cesarean Delivery at 37 Weeks of Gestation or Greater with Singleton Fetuses with Vertex Presentations—VBAC*
Alabama	20.4	23.3
Alaska	16.1	36.9
Arizona	13.4	31.6
Arkansas	21.8	20.4
California	18.1	24.3
Colorado	12.3	44.2
Connecticut	16.8	37.1
Delaware	17.1	36.4
District of Columbia	21.6	22.7
Florida	18.7	27.5
Georgia	18.1	26.8
Hawaii	15.0	37.1
Idaho	11.8	39.1
Illinois	16.5	32.8
Indiana	18.1	27.9
Iowa	15.3	38.4
Kansas	16.0	27.0
Kentucky	18.0	28.7
Louisiana	24.2	13.6
Maine	17.2	33.2
Maryland	20.6	35.4
Massachusetts	17.1	36.4
Michigan	16.9	28.7
Minnesota	13.9	39.3
Mississippi	24.3	18.7
Missouri	16.9	34.3
Montana	16.0	36.4
Nebraska	16.4	33.4
Nevada	16.8	30.7
New Hampshire	18.6	34.3
New Jersey	20.9	37.6
New Mexico	13.3	40.3
New York	20.4	33.0
North Carolina	18.6	30.9
North Dakota	15.9	31.3
Ohio	15.7	38.2
Oklahoma	18.7	23.3
Oregon	14.5	42.2
Pennsylvania	16.6	37.1
Rhode Island	16.2	38.7
South Carolina	19.7	24.5
South Dakota	17.4	25.7
Tennessee	19.4	29.0
Texas	20.0	23.2
Utah	11.5	37.1
Vermont	15.3	43.2
Virginia	19.0	34.3
Washington	14.0	38.3
West Virginia	18.3	25.5
Wisconsin	13.9	36.5
Wyoming	15.0	36.8

* Abbreviation: VBAC, vaginal birth after cesarean delivery.

References

1. Miller JM Jr. Maternal and neonatal morbidity and mortality in cesarean section. Obstet Gynecol Clin North Am 1988;15:629–638 (III)

2. Sachs BP, Yeh J, Acker D, Driscoll S, Brown DA, Jewett JF. Cesarean section-related maternal mortality in Massachusetts, 1954–1985. Obstet Gynecol 1988;71:385–388 (II-3)

3. Depp R. Cesarean delivery. In Gabbe SG, Neibyl JR, Simpson JL, eds. Obstetrics normal and problem pregnancies. Churchill Livingstone, New York, 1996:561–642 (III)

4. Durfee R. Cesarean section. In Nichols DH, ed. Gynecologic and obstetric surgery. St. Louis, Missouri: Mosby-Year Book, 1993:1075–1122 (III)

5. Stedman CM, Kline RC. Intraoperative complications and unexpected pathology at the time of cesarean section. Obstet Gynecol Clin North Am 1988;15:745–769 (III)

6. Nielsen TF, Hokegard KH. Cesarean section and intraoperative surgical complications. Acta Obstet Gynecol Scand 1984;63:103–108 (II-3)

7. Chazotte C, Cohen WR. Catastrophic complications of previous cesarean section. Am J Obstet Gynecol 1990;163:738–742 (III)

8. Resnik R. Diagnosis and management of placenta accreta. ACOG Clinical Review 1999;4(2):8–9 (III)

9. American Academy of Pediatrics, American College of Obstetricians and Gynecologists. Guidelines for perinatal care. 4th ed. Elk Grove Village, Illinois: AAP; Washington: ACOG, 1997 (III)

10. Owen J, Andrews WW. Wound complications after cesarean sections. Clin Obstet Gynecol 1994;37:842–855 (III)

11. Webster J. Post-caesarean wound infection: a review of the risk factors. Aust N Z J Obstet Gynaecol 1988;28:201–207 (II-3)

12. Ananth CV, Smulian JC, Vintzileos AM. The association of placenta previa with history of cesarean delivery and abortion: a meta-analysis. Am J Obstet Gynecol 1997;177:1071–1078 (Meta-analysis)

13. Hershkowitz R, Fraser D, Mazor M, Leiberman JR. One or multiple previous cesarean sections are associated with similar increased frequency of placenta previa. Eur J Obstet Gynecol Reprod Biol 1995;62:185–188 (II-3)

14. Clark SL, Koonings PP, Phelan JP. Placenta previa/accreta and prior cesarean section. Obstet Gynecol 1985;66:89–92 (II-3)

15. Nielsen TF, Hagberg H, Ljungblad U. Placenta previa and antepartum hemorrhage after previous cesarean section. Gynecol Obstet Invest 1989;27:88–90 (II-3)

16. Taylor VM, Kramer MD, Vaughan TL, Peacock S. Placenta previa and prior cesarean delivery: how strong is the association? Obstet Gynecol 1994;84:55–57 (II-2)

17. McMahon MJ, Li R, Schenck AP, Olshan AF, Royce RA. Previous cesarean birth. A risk factor for placenta previa? J Reprod Med 1997;42:409–412 (II-2)

18. Chattopadhyay SK, Kharif H, Sherbeeni MM. Placenta praevia and accreta after previous caesarean section. Eur J Obstet Gynecol Reprod Biol 1993;52:151–156 (II-3)

19. Stanco LM, Schrimmer DB, Paul RH, Mishell DR Jr. Emergency peripartum hysterectomy and associated risk factors. Am J Obstet Gynecol 1993;168:879–883 (II-3)

20. Manyonda IT, Varma TR. Massive obstetric hemorrhage due to placenta previa/accreta with prior cesarean section. Int J Gynaecol Obstet 1990;34:183–186 (III)

21. National Center for Health Statistics. Infant deaths and infant mortality rates by method of delivery, age and race of mother: United States, 1995. Washington: Centers for Disease Control and Prevention, 1999 (II-3)

22. Shearer EL. Cesarean section: medical benefits and costs. Soc Sci Med 1993;37:1223–1231 (III)

23. Handa VL, Harris TA, Ostergard DR. Protecting the pelvic floor: obstetric management to prevent incontinence and pelvic organ prolapse. Obstet Gynecol 1996;88:470–478 (III)

24. Meyer S, de Grandi P, Kuntzer T, Hurlimann P, Schmidt N. Birth trauma: its effect on the urine continence mechanisms. Gynakol Geburtshilfliche Rundsch 1993;33:236–242 (III)

25. Peschers U, Schaer G, Anthuber C, Delancey JO, Schuessler B. Changes in vesical neck mobility following vaginal delivery. Obstet Gynecol 1996;88:1001–1006 (II-2)

26. Ryhammer AM, Laurberg S, Hermann AP. Long-term effect of vaginal deliveries on anorectal function in normal perimenopausal women. Dis Colon Rectum 1996;39:852–859 (II-3)

27. Deindl FM, Vodusek DB, Hesse U, Schussler B. Pelvic floor activity patterns: comparison of nulliparous continent and parous urinary stress incontinent women. A kinesiological EMG study. Br J Urol 1994;73:413–417 (II-2)

28. Snooks SJ, Swash M, Henry MM, Setchell M. Risk factors in childbirth causing damage to the pelvic floor innervation. Int J Colorectal Dis 1986;1:20–24 (II-2)

29. Sultan AH, Kamm MA, Hudson CN. Pudendal nerve damage during labour: prospective study before and after childbirth. Br J Obstet Gynaecol 1994;101:22–28 (II-2)

30. Sultan AH, Kamm MA, Hudson CN, Thomas JM, Bartram CI. Anal-sphincter disruption during vaginal delivery. N Engl J Med 1993;329:1905–1911 (II-3)

31. Ryhammer AM, Bek KM, Laurberg S. Multiple vaginal deliveries increase the risk of permanent incontinence of flatus and urine in normal premenopausal women. Dis Colon Rectum 1995;38:1206–1209 (II-3)

32. Sultan AH, Kamm MA, Hudson CN, Bartram CI. Third degree obstetric anal sphincter tears: risk factors and outcome of primary repair. BMJ 1994;308:887–891 (II-2)

33. MacArthur C, Bick DE, Keighley MR. Faecal incontinence after childbirth. Br J Obstet Gynaecol 1997;104:46–50 (II-2)

34. Fornell EK, Berg G, Hallböök O, Matthiesen LS, Sjodahl R. Clinical consequences of anal sphincter rupture during vaginal delivery. J Am Coll Surg 1996:183:553–558 (II-2)

35. Crawford LA, Quint EH, Pearl ML, DeLancey JO. Incontinence following rupture of the anal sphincter during delivery. Obstet Gynecol 1993;82:527–531 (II-2)

36. Walsh CJ, Mooney EF, Upton GJ, Motson RW. Incidence of third-degree perineal tears in labour and outcome after primary repair. Br J Surg 1996;83:218–221 (II-3)

37. Tetzschner T, Sorensen M, Lose G, Christiansen J. Anal and urinary incontinence in women with obstetric anal sphincter rupture. Br J Obstet Gynaecol 1996;103:1034–1040 (II-3)

38. Wilson PD, Herbison RM, Herbison GP. Obstetric practice and the prevalence of urinary incontinence three months after delivery. Br J Obstet Gynaecol 1996;103:154–161 (II-3)

39. Smith AR, Hosker GL, Warrell DW. The role of pudendal nerve damage in the aetiology of genuine stress incontinence in women. Br J Obstet Gynaecol 1989;96:29–32 (II-2)

40. Röckner G. Urinary incontinence after perineal trauma at childbirth. Scand J Caring Sci 1990;4:169–172 (II-3)

41. Skoner MM, Thompson WD, Caron VA. Factors associated with risk of stress urinary incontinence in women. Nurs Res 1994;43:301–306 (II-2)

42. Sultan AH, Stanton SL. Preserving the pelvic floor and perineum during childbirth—elective caesarean section? Br J Obstet Gynaecol 1996;103:731–734 (III)

43. Taffel SM. Cesarean delivery in the United States, 1990. Vital Health Stat 21 1994;51:1–24 (II-3)

44. Ventura SJ, Martin JA, Curtin SC, Mathews TJ. Birth: final data for 1997. Natl Vital Stat Rep 1999;47:1–83 (II-3)

45. Clarke SC, Taffel SM. Rates of cesarean and VBAC delivery, United States, 1994. Birth 1996;23:166–168 (II-3)

46. Clarke SC, Taffel S. Changes in cesarean delivery in the United States, 1988 and 1993. Birth 1995;22:63–67 (II-3)

47. McKenzie L, Stephenson PA. Variation in cesarean section rates among hospitals in Washington state. Am J Public Health 1993;83:1109–1112 (II-3)

48. Taffel SM. Cesarean section in America: dramatic trends, 1970 to 1987. Stat Bull Metrop Insur Co 1989;70:2–11

49. Hueston WJ. Site-to-site variation in the factors affecting cesarean section rates. Arch Fam Med 1995;4:346–351 (II-2)

50. Lieberman E. Predictors of cesarean delivery. Curr Probl Obstet Gynecol Fertil 1997;20:98–131 (III)

51. Sanchez-Ramos L, Moorhead RI, Kaunitz AM. Cesarean section rates in teaching hospitals: a national survey. Birth 1994;21:194–196 (II-3)

52. Tussing AD, Wojtowycz MA. The cesarean decision in New York State, 1986. Economic and noneconomic aspects. Med Care 1992;30:529–540 (II-2)

53. Carpenter MW, Soule D, Yates WT, Meeker CI. Practice environment is associated with obstetric decision making regarding abnormal labor. Obstet Gynecol 1987;70:657–662 (II-2)

54. Klasko SK, Cummings RV, Balducci J, DeFulvio JD, Reed JF 3rd. The impact of mandated in-hospital coverage on primary cesarean delivery rates in a large nonuniversity teaching hospital. Am J Obstet Gynecol 1995;172:637–642 (II-2)

55. DeMott RK, Sandmire HF. The Green Bay cesarean section study. II. The physician factor as a determinant of cesarean birth rates for failed labor. Am J Obstet Gynecol 1992;166:1799–1806; discussion 1806–1810 (II-2)

56. Socol ML, Peaceman AM Vaginal birth after cesarean: an appraisal of fetal risk. Obstet Gynecol 1999;93:674–679 (II-2)

57. Tussing AD, Wojtowycz MA. The effect of physician characteristics on clinical behavior: cesarean section in New York State. Soc Sci Med 1993;37:1251–1260 (II-3)

58. Radin TG. Harmon JS, Hanson DA. Nurses' care during labor: its effect on the cesarean birth rate of healthy, nulliparous women. Birth 1993;20:14–21 (II-3)

59. Brown HS. Physician demand for leisure: implications for cesarean section rates. J Health Econ 1996;15:233–242 (II-3)

60. Phillips RN, Thornton J, Gleicher N. Physician bias in cesarean sections. JAMA 1982;248:1082–1084 (II-3)

61. Goyert GL, Bottoms SF, Treadwell MC, Nehra PC. The physician factor in cesarean birth rates. N Engl J Med 1989:320:706–709 (II-3)

62. McCloskey L, Petitti DB, Hobel CJ. Variations in the use of cesarean delivery for dystocia: lessons about the source of care. Med Care 1992;30:126–135 (II-2)

63. Bertollini R, DiLallo D, Spadea T, Perucci C. Cesarean section rates in Italy by hospital payment mode: an analysis based on birth certificates. Am J Public Health 1992;82:257–261 (II-2)

64. Tussing AD, Wojtowycz MA. Health maintenance organizations, independent practice associations, and cesarean section rates. Health Serv Res 1994;29:75–93 (II-3)

65. Stafford RS. The impact of nonclinical factors on repeat cesarean section. JAMA 1991;265:59–63 (II-2)

66. Price MR, Broomberg J. The impact of the fee-for-service reimbursement system on the utilisation of health services. Part III. A comparison of caesarean section rates in white nulliparous women in the private and public sectors. S Afr Med J 1990;78:136–138 (II-2)

67. Stafford RS. Cesarean section use and source of payment: an analysis of California hospital discharge abstracts. Am J Public Health 1990;80:313–315 (II-2)

68. Newton ER, Higgins CS. Factors associated with hospital-specific cesarean birth rates. J Reprod Med 1989;34:407–411 (II-3)

69. Gould JB, Davey B, Stafford RS. Socioeconomic differences in rates of cesarean section. N Engl J Med 1989;321:233–239 (II-2)

70. Braveman P, Egerter S, Edmonston F, Verdon M. Racial/ethnic differences in the likelihood of cesarean delivery, California. Am J Public Health 1995;85:625–630 (II-2)

71. King DE, Lahiri K. Socioeconomic factors and the odds of vaginal birth after cesarean delivery. JAMA 1994;272:524–529 (II-2)

72. Hodnett E. Nursing support of the laboring woman. J Obstet Gynecol Neonatal Nurs 1996;25:257–264 (III)

73. McNiven P, Hodnett E, O'Brien-Pallas L. Supporting women in labor: a work sampling study of the activities of labor and delivery nurses. Birth 1992;19:3–9 (III)

74. Gagnon AJ, Waghorn K. Supportive care by maternity nurses: a work sampling study in an intrapartum unit. Birth 1996;23:1–6 (III)

75. Frigoletto FD Jr, Lieberman E, Lang JM, Cohen A, Barss V, Ringer S, et al. A clinical trial of active management of labor. N Engl J Med 1995;333:745–750 (I) [published erratum appears in N Engl J Med 1997;333:1163]

76. Gagnon AJ, Waghorn K, Covell C. A randomized trial of one-to-one nurse support of women in labor. Birth 1997;24:71–77 (I)

77. Zhang J, Bernasko JW, Leybovich E, Fahs M, Hatch MC. Continuous labor support from labor attendant for primiparous women: a meta-analysis. Obstet Gynecol 1996;88:739–744 (Meta-analysis)

78. Hodnett E. Caregiver support for women during childbirth (Cochrane review). In: The Cochrane Library, Issue 3, 1999. Oxford: Update Software (Meta-analysis)

79. Hodnett E. Commentary: are nurses effective providers of labor support? Should they be? Can they be? Birth 1997;24:78–80 (III)

80. Stanley FJ, Watson L. Trends in perinatal mortality and cerebral palsy in Western Australia, 1967 to 1985. BMJ 1992;304:1658–1663 (II-3)

81. Nelson KB, Dambrosia JM, Ting TY, Grether JK. Uncertain value of electronic fetal monitoring in predicting cerebral palsy. N Engl J Med 1996;334:613–618 (II-2)

82. American College of Obstetricians and Gynecologists. Inappropriate use of the terms fetal distress and birth asphyxia. ACOG Committee Opinion 197. Washington: ACOG, 1998 (III)

83. Tussing AD, Wojtowycz MA. Malpractice, defensive medicine, and obstetric behavior. Med Care 1997;35:172–191 (II-3)

84. Savage W, Francome C. British caesarean section rates: have we reached a plateau? Br J Obstet Gynaecol 1993;100:493–496 (II-3)

85. Rock SM. Malpractice premiums and primary cesarean section rates in New York and Illinois. Public Health Rep 1988;103:459–463 (III)

86. Localio AR, Lawthers AG, Bengston JM, Hebert LE, Weaver SL, Brennan TA, et al. Relationship between malpractice claims and cesarean delivery. JAMA 1993:269:366–373 (II-3)

87. Griffin LP, Heland KV, Esser L, Jones S. Overview of the 1996 Professional Liability Survey. ACOG Clinical Review 1998;3:1–2, 13–14 (II-3)

88. Ventura SJ. Trends and variations in first births to older women, United States, 1970–86. Vital Health Stat 21 1989;47:1–27 (II-3)

89. Morrison I. The elderly primigravida. Am J Obstet Gynecol 1975;121:465–470 (II-2)

90. Blum M. Is the elderly primipara really at high risk? J Perinat Med 1979;7:108–112 (II-2)

91. Kessler I, Lancet M, Borenstein R, Steinmetz A. The problem of the older primipara. Obstet Gynecol 1980;56:165–169 (II-2)

92. Grimes DA, Gross GK. Pregnancy outcomes in black women aged 35 and older. Obstet Gynecol 1981;58:614–620 (II-2)

93. Kirz DS, Dorchester W, Freeman RK. Advanced maternal age: the mature gravida. Am J Obstet Gynecol 1985;152:7–12 (II-2)

94. Martel M, Wacholder S, Lippman A, Brohan J, Hamilton E. Maternal age and primary cesarean section rates: a multivariate analysis. Am J Obstet Gynecol 1987;156:305–308 (II-2)

95. Tuck SM, Yudkin PL, Turnbull AC. Pregnancy outcome in elderly primigravidae with and without a history of infertility. Br J Obstet Gynaecol 1988;95:230–237 (II-2)

96. Gordon D, Milberg J, Daling J, Hickok D. Advanced maternal age as a risk factor for cesarean delivery. Obstet Gynecol 1991;77:493–497 (II-2)

97. Peipert JF, Bracken MB. Maternal age: an independent risk factor for cesarean delivery. Obstet Gynecol 1993;81:200–205 (II-2)

98. Adashek JA, Peaceman AM, Lopez-Zeno JA, Minogue JP, Socol ML. Factors contributing to the increased cesarean birth rate in older parturient women. Am J Obstet Gynecol 1993;169:936–940 (II-2)

99. Edge V, Laros RK Jr. Pregnancy outcome in nulliparous women aged 35 or older. Am J Obstet Gynecol 1993;168:1881–1885 (II-2)

100. Vercellini P, Zuliani G, Rognoni MT, Trespidi L, Oldani S, Cardinale A. Pregnancy at forty and over: a case-control study. Eur J Obstet Gynecol Reprod Biol 1993;48:191–195 (II-2)

101. Parrish KM, Holt VL, Easterling TR, Connell FA, LoGerfo JP. Effect of changes in maternal age, parity, and birth weight distribution on primary cesarean delivery rates. JAMA 1994;271:443–447 (II-2)

102. Bobrowski RA, Bottoms SF. Underappreciated risks of the elderly multipara. Am J Obstet Gynecol 1995;172:1764–1770 (II-2)

103. Prysak M, Lorenz RP, Kisly A. Pregnancy outcome in nulliparous women 35 years and older. Obstet Gynecol 1995;85:65–70 (II-2)

104. Bianco A, Stone J, Lynch L, Lapinski R, Berkowitz G, Berkowitz RL. Pregnancy outcome at age 40 and older. Obstet Gynecol 1996;87:917–922 (II-2)

105. Brassil MJ, Turner MJ, Egan DM, MacDonald DW. Obstetric outcome in first-time mothers aged 40 years and over. Eur J Obstet Gynecol Reprod Biol 1987;25:115–120 (II-2)

106. Dollberg S, Seidman DS, Armon Y, Stevenson DK, Gale R. Adverse perinatal outcome in the older primipara. J Perinatol 1996;16:93–97 (II-2)

107. Scholl TO, Hediger ML, Belsky DH. Prenatal care and maternal health during adolescent pregnancy: a review and meta-analysis. J Adolesc Health 1994;15:444–456 (Meta-analysis)

108. Berkowitz GS, Skovron ML, Lapinski RH, Berkowitz RL. Delayed childbearing and the outcome of pregnancy. N Engl J Med 1990;322:659–664 (II-2)

109. Waters EG, Wager HP. Pregnancy and labor experiences of elderly primigravidas. Am J Obstet Gynecol 1950;59:296–304 (II-2)

110. Cunningham FG, Leveno KJ. Childbearing among older women—the message is cautiously optimistic. N Engl J Med 1995;333:1002–1004 (II-2)

111. Johnson JW, Longmate JA, Frentzen B. Excessive maternal weight and pregnancy outcome. Am J Obstet Gynecol 1992;167:353–372 (II-2)

112. Harlow BL, Frigoletto FD, Cramer DW, Evans JK, Bain RP, Ewigman B, et al. Epidemiologic predictors of cesarean section in nulliparous patients at low risk. RADIUS Study Group. Routine Antenatal Diagnostic Imaging with Ultrasound Study. Am J Obstet Gynecol 1995;172:156–162 (II-3)

113. Edwards LE, Dickes WF, Alton IR, Hakanson EY. Pregnancy in the massively obese: course, outcome, and obesity prognosis of the infant. Am J Obstet Gynecol 1978;131:479–483 (II-2)

114. Gross T, Sokol RJ, King KC. Obesity in pregnancy: risks and outcome. Obstet Gynecol 1980;56:446–450 (II-2)

115. Garbaciak JA Jr, Richter M, Miller S, Barton JJ. Maternal weight and pregnancy complications. Am J Obstet Gynecol 1985;152:238–245 (II-2)

116. Johnson SR, Kolberg BH, Varner MW, Railsback LD. Maternal obesity and pregnancy. Surg Gynecol Obstet 1987;164:431–437 (II-2)

117. Perlow JH, Morgan MA, Montgomery D, Towers CV, Porto M. Perinatal outcome in pregnancy complicated by massive obesity. Am J Obstet Gynecol 1992;167:958–962 (II-2)

118. Crane SS, Wojtowycz MA, Dye TD, Aubry RH, Artal R. Association between pre-pregnancy obesity and the risk of cesarean delivery. Obstet Gynecol 1997;89:213–216 (II-2)

119. Brost BC, Goldenberg RL, Mercer BM, Iams JD, Meis PJ, Moawad AH, et al. The Preterm Prediction Study: association of cesarean delivery with increases in maternal weight and body mass index. Am J Obstet Gynecol 1997;177:333–341 (II-2)

120. Witter FR, Caulfield LE, Stoltzfus RJ. Influence of maternal anthropometric status and birth weight on the risk of cesarean delivery. Obstet Gynecol 1995;85:947–951 (II-2)

121. Kuczmarski RJ, Flegal KM, Campbell SM, Johnson CL. Increasing prevalence of overweight among US adults. The National Health and Nutrition Examination Surveys, 1960 to 1991. JAMA 1994;272:205–211 (II-3)

122. Ramin SM, Cunningham FG. Obesity in pregnancy. In: Cunningham FG, ed. Williams obstetrics. 19th ed. Supplement No. 13. Norwalk, Connecticut: Appleton & Lange, 1995 (III)

123. Institute of Medicine, Subcommittee on Nutritional Status and Weight Gain During Pregnancy. Nutrition during pregnancy. Part 1: weight gain. Washington: National Academy Press, 1990 (III)

124. American College of Obstetricians and Gynecologists. Vaginal birth after previous cesarean delivery. ACOG Practice Bulletin 5. Washington, DC: ACOG, 1999 (III)

125. Notzon FC, Cnattingius S, Bergsjo P, Cole S, Taffel S, Irgens L, et al. Cesarean section delivery in the 1980s: international comparison by indication. Am J Obstet Gynecol 1994;170:495–504 (II-3)

126. Paul RH, Miller DA. Cesarean birth: how to reduce the rate. Am J Obstet Gynecol 1995;172:1903–1911 (III)

127. Rosen MG, Dickinson JC, Westhoff CL. Vaginal birth after cesarean: a meta-analysis of morbidity and mortality. Obstet Gynecol 1991;77:465–470 (Meta-analysis)

128. Flamm BL. Vaginal birth after cesarean section. In: Flamm BL, Quilligan EJ, eds. Cesarean section: guidelines for appropriate utilization. New York: Springer-Verlag, 1995:51–64 (III)

129. Pridjian G. Labor after prior cesarean section. Clin Obstet Gynecol 1992;35:445–456 (III)

130. Bedoya C, Bartha JL, Rodriguez I, Fontan I, Bedoya JM, Sanchez-Ramos J. A trial of labor after cesarean section in patients with or without a prior vaginal delivery. Int J Gynaecol Obstet 1992;39:285–289 (II-2)

131. Eglinton GS. Effect of previous indications for cesarean on subsequent outcome. In: Phelan JP, Clark SL, eds. Cesarean delivery. New York: Elsevier,1988:476–483 (III)

132. Leung AS, Farmer RM, Leung EK, Medearis AL, Paul RH. Risk factors associated with uterine rupture during trial of labor after cesarean delivery: a case-control study. Am J Obstet Gynecol 1993;168:1358–1363 (II-2)

133. Flamm BL, Goings JR, Lin Y, Wolde-Tsadik G. Elective repeat cesarean delivery versus trial of labor: a prospective multicenter study. Obstet Gynecol 1994;83:927–932 (II-2)

134. McMahon MJ, Luther ER, Bowes WA Jr, Olshan AF. Comparison of a trial of labor with an elective

second cesarean section. N Engl J Med 1996;335: 689–695 (II-2)

135. Scott JR. Mandatory trial of labor after cesarean delivery: an alternative viewpoint. Obstet Gynecol 1991;77:811–814 (III)

136. Jones RO, Nagashima AW, Hartnett-Goodman MM, Goodlin RC. Rupture of low transverse cesarean scars during trial of labor. Obstet Gynecol 1991;77: 815–817 (III)

137. Porter TF, Clark SL, Esplin MS, Tooke-Miller C, Scott JR. Timing of delivery and neonatal outcome in patients with clinically overt uterine rupture during VBAC. SPO Abstract #73. Am J Obstet Gynecol 1998;178:S31

138. Farmer RM, Kirschbaum T, Potter D, Strong TH, Medearis AL. Uterine rupture during trial of labor after previous cesarean section. Am J Obstet Gynecol 1991;165:996–1001 (II-2)

139. Fraser W, Maunsell E, Hodnett E, Moutquin JM. Randomized controlled trial of a prenatal vaginal birth after cesarean section education and support program. Childbirth Alternatives Post-Cesarean Study Group. Am J Obstet Gynecol 1997;176: 419–425 (II-1)

140. Goldman G, Pineault R, Potvin L, Blais R, Bilodeau H. Factors influencing the practice of vaginal birth after cesarean section. Am J Public Health 1993; 83:1104–1108 (II-2)

141. Lomas J, Enkin M, Anderson GM, Hannah WJ, Vayda E, Singer J. Opinion leaders vs audit and feedback to implement practice guidelines. Delivery after previous cesarean section. JAMA 1991;265:2202–2207 (I)

142. Lagrew DC Jr, Morgan MA. Decreasing the cesarean section rate in a private hospital: success without mandated clinical changes. Am J Obstet Gynecol 1996;174:184–191 (II-2)

143. Poma PA. Effect of departmental policies on cesarean delivery rates: a community hospital experience. Obstet Gynecol 1998;91:1013–1018 (II-2)

144. Ventura SJ, Martin JA, Curtin SC, Mathews TJ. Report of final natality statistics, 1996. Mon Vital Stat Rep 1998;46(11 Suppl):1–99 (II-3)

145. Menticoglou SM, Manning F, Harmon C, Morrison I. Perinatal outcome in relation to second stage duration. Am J Obstet Gynecol 1995;173:906–912 (II-3)

146. National Maternity Hospital. Clinical report for the year 1992. Dublin: NMH, 1992 (III)

147. Turner MJ, Brassil M, Gordon H. Active management of labor associated with a decrease in the cesarean section rate in nulliparas. Obstet Gynecol 1988;71:150–154 (II-3)

148. Akoury HA, Brodie G, Caddick R, McLaughlin VD, Pugh PA. Active management of labor and operative delivery in nulliparous women. Am J Obstet Gynecol 1988;158:255–258 (II-2)

149. Boylan P, Frankowski R, Rountree R, Selwyn B, Parrish K. Effect of active management of labor on the incidence of cesarean section for dystocia in nulliparas. Am J Perinatol 1991;8:373–379 (II-2)

150. Lopez-Zeno JA, Peaceman AM, Adashek JA, Socol ML. A controlled trial of a program for the active management of labor. N Engl J Med 1992;326: 450–454 (I)

151. Thorp JA, Parisi VM, Boylan PC, Johnston DA. The effect of continuous epidural analgesia on cesarean section for dystocia in nulliparous women. Am J Obstet Gynecol 1989;161:670–675 (II-2)

152. Thorp JA, Eckert LO, Ang MS, Johnston DA, Peaceman AM, Parisi VM. Epidural analgesia and cesarean section for dystocia: risk factors in nulliparas. Am J Perinatol 1991;8:402–410 (II-2)

153. Peaceman AM, Lopez-Zeno JA, Minogue JP, Socol ML. Factors that influence route of delivery— active versus traditional labor management. Am J Obstet Gynecol 1993;169:940–944 (I)

154. Gribble RK, Meier PR. Effect of epidural analgesia on the primary cesarean rate. Obstet Gynecol 1991;78:231–234 (II-2)

155. Lieberman E, Lang JM, Cohen A, D'Agostino R Jr, Datta S, Frigoletto FD Jr. Association of epidural analgesia with cesarean delivery in nulliparas. Obstet Gynecol 1996;88:993–1000 (II-2)

156. Philipsen T, Jensen NH. Epidural block or parenteral pethidine as analgesic in labour; a randomized study concerning progress in labour and instrumental deliveries. Eur J Obstet Gynecol Reprod Biol 1989;30:27–33 (I)

157. Thorp JA, Hu DH, Albin RM, McNitt J, Meyer BA, Cohen GR, et al. The effect of intrapartum epidural analgesia on nulliparous labor: a randomized, controlled, prospective trial. Am J Obstet Gynecol 1993;169:851–858 (I)

158. Ramin SM, Gambling DR, Lucas MJ, Sharma SK, Sidawi JE, Leveno KJ. Randomized trial of epidural versus intravenous analgesia during labor. Obstet Gynecol 1995;86:783–789 (II-1)

159. Sharma SK, Sidawi JE, Ramin SM, Lucas MJ, Leveno KJ, Cunningham FG. Cesarean delivery: a randomized trial of epidural versus patient-controlled meperidine analgesia during labor. Anesthesiology 1997;87:487–494 (I)

160. Nageotte MP, Larson D, Rumney PJ, Sidhu M, Hollenbach K. Epidural analgesia compared with combined spinal-epidural analgesia during labor in nulliparous women. New Engl J Med 1997;337: 1715–1719 (II-1)

161. Chestnut DH, McGrath JM, Vincent RD Jr, Penning DH, Choi WW, Bates JN, et al. Does early administration of epidural analgesia affect obstetric outcome in nulliparous women who are in spontaneous labor? Anesthesiology 1994;80:1201–1206 (I)

162. Bofill JA, Vincent RD, Ross EL, Martin RW, Norman PF, Werhan CF, et al. Nulliparous active labor, epidural analgesia, and cesarian delivery for dystocia. Am J Obstet Gynecol 1997;177: 1465–1470 (I)

163. Kelly VC, Kulkarni D. Experiences with fetal monitoring in a community hospital. Obstet Gynecol 1973;4:818–824 (III)

164. Paul RH, Hon EH. Clinical fetal monitoring. V. Effect on perinatal outcome. Am J Obstet Gynecol 1974;118:529–533 (II-3)

165. Haverkamp AD, Thompson HE, McFee JG, Cetrulo C. The evaluation of continuous fetal heart rate monitoring in high-risk pregnancy. Am J Obstet Gynecol 1976;125:310–320 (I)

166. Kelso IM, Parsons RJ, Lawrence GF, Arora SS, Edmonds DK, Cooke ID. An assessment of continuous fetal heart rate monitoring in labor. A randomized trial. Am J Obstet Gynecol 1978;131:526–532 (I)

167. Haverkamp AD, Orleans M, Langendoerfer S, McFee J, Murphy J, Thompson HE. A controlled trial of the differential effects of intrapartum fetal monitoring. Am J Obstet Gynecol 1979;134: 399–412 (I)

168. Wood C, Renou P, Oates J, Farrell E, Beischer N, Anderson I. A controlled trial of fetal heart rate monitoring in a low-risk obstetric population. Am J Obstet Gynecol 1981;141:527–534 (II-1)

169. Neldam S, Osler M, Hansen PK, Nim J, Smith SF, Hertel J. Intrapartum fetal heart rate monitoring in a combined low- and high-risk population: a controlled clinical trial. Eur J Obstet Gynecol Reprod Biol 1986;23:1–11 (I)

170. MacDonald D, Grant A, Sheridan-Pereira M, Boylan P, Chalmers I. The Dublin randomized controlled trial of intrapartum fetal heart rate monitoring. Am J Obstet Gynecol 1985;152:524–539 (I)

171. Luthy DA, Shy KK, van Belle G, Larson EB, Hughes JP, Benedetti TJ, et al. A randomized trial of electronic fetal monitoring in preterm labor. Obstet Gynecol 1987;69:687–695 (I)

172. Thacker SB, Stroup DF, Peterson HB. Efficacy and safety of intrapartum electronic fetal monitoring: an update. Obstet Gynecol 1995;86:613–620 (III)

173. Freeman R. Intrapartum fetal monitoring—a disappointing story. N Engl J Med 1990;322:624–626 (III)

174. Schifrin B, Dame L. Fetal heart rate patterns. Prediction of Apgar score. JAMA 1972;219: 1322–1325 (II-3)

175. Hon EH, Khazin AF, Paul RH. Biochemical studies of the fetus. II. Fetal pH and apgar scores. Obstet Gynecol 1969;33:237–255 (II-3)

176. Miyazaki F, Nevarez F. Saline amnioinfusion for relief of repetitive variable decelerations: a prospective randomized study. Am J Obstet Gynecol 1985; 153:301–306 (I)

177. Nageotte MP, Freeman RK, Garite TJ, Dorchester W. Prophylactic intrapartum amnioinfusion in patients with preterm premature rupture of membranes. Am J Obstet Gynecol 1985;153:557–562 (I)

178. Macri CJ, Schrimmer DB, Leung A, Greenspoon JS, Paul RH. Prophylactic amnioinfusion improves outcome of pregnancy complicated by thick meconium and oligohydramnios. Am J Obstet Gynecol 1992;167:117–121 (I)

179. American College of Obstetricians and Gynecologists. Fetal heart rate patterns: monitoring, interpretation, and management. ACOG Educational Bulletin 207. Washington: ACOG, 1995 (III)

180. Tejani N, Mann LI, Bhakthavathsalan A. Correlation with fetal heart rate patterns and fetal pH with neonatal outcome. Obstet Gynecol 1976;48: 460–463 (II-3)

181. Clark SL, Gimovsky ML, Miller FC. The scalp stimulation test: a clinical alternative to fetal scalp blood sampling. Am J Obstet Gynecol 1984;148: 274–277 (II-3)

182. American College of Obstetricians and Gynecologists. Shoulder dystocia. ACOG Practice Pattern 7. Washington: ACOG, 1997 (III)

183. Levine AB, Lockwood CJ, Brown B, Lapinski R, Berkowitz RL. Sonographic diagnosis of the large for gestational age fetus at term: does it make a difference? Obstet Gynecol 1992;79:55–58 (II-3)

184. Weeks JW, Pitman T, Spinnato JA 2nd. Fetal macrosomia: does antenatal prediction affect delivery route and birth outcome? Am J Obstet Gynecol 1995;173:1215–1219 (II-2)

185. Delpapa EH, Mueller-Heubach E. Pregnancy outcome following ultrasound diagnosis of macrosomia. Obstet Gynecol 1991;78:340–343 (II-3)

186. Hedriana HL, Moore TR. A comparison of single versus multiple growth ultrasonographic examinations in predicting birth weight. Am J Obstet Gynecol 1994;170:1600–1606 (II-3)

187. Bernstein IM, Catalano PM. Influence of fetal fat on the ultrasound estimation of fetal weight in diabetic mothers. Obstet Gynecol 1992;79:561–563 (II-3)

189. Leaphart WL, Meyer MC, Capeless EL. Labor induction with a prenatal diagnosis of fetal macrosomia. J Matern Fetal Med 1997;6:99–102 (II-2)

190. Diani F, Moscatelli C, Toppano B, Turinetto A. Fetal macrosomia and mode of delivery. Minerva Ginecol 1995;47:77–82 (II-3)

191. Combs CA, Singh NB, Khoury JC. Elective induction versus spontaneous labor after sonographic diagnosis of fetal macrosomia. Obstet Gynecol 1993;81:492–496 (II-2)

192. Gonen O, Rosen DJ, Dolfin Z, Tepper R, Markov S, Fejgin MD. Induction of labor versus expectant management in macrosomia: a randomized study. Obstet Gynecol 1997;89:913–917 (I)

193. American College of Obstetricians and Gynecologists. Induction of labor. ACOG Practice Bulletin 10. Washington: ACOG, 1999 (III)

194. Ingemarsson I, Kallen K. Stillbirths and rate of neonatal deaths in 76,761 postterm pregnancies in Sweden, 1982–1991: a register study. Acta Obstet Gynecol Scand 1997;76:658–662 (II-2)

195. American College of Obstetricians and Gynecologists. Management of postterm pregnancy. ACOG Practice Pattern 6. Washington: ACOG, 1997 (III)

196. Hannah ME, Huh C, Hewson SA, Hannah WJ. Postterm pregnancy: putting the merits of a policy of induction of labor into perspective. Birth 1996;23:13–19 (I)

197. Goeree R, Hannah M, Hewson S. Cost-effectiveness of induction of labour versus serial antenatal monitoring in the Canadian Multicentre Postterm Pregnancy Trial. CMAJ 1995;152:1445–1450 (Cost-effectiveness analysis)

198. National Institute of Child Health and Human Development Network of Maternal-Fetal Medicine Units. A clinical trial of induction of labor versus expectant management in postterm pregnancy. Am J Obstet Gynecol 1994;170:716–723 (I)

199. Roman J, Bakos O, Cnattingus S. Pregnancy outcomes by mode of delivery among term breech births: Swedish experience 1987–1993. Obstet Gynecol 1998;92:945–950 (II-2)

200. Stine LE, Phelan JP, Wallace R, Eglinton GS, van Dorsten JP, Schifrin BS. Update on external cephalic version performed at term. Obstet Gynecol 1985;65:642–646 (III)

201. Eller DP, VanDorsten JP. Route of delivery for the breech presentation: a conundrum. Am J Obstet Gynecol 1995;173:393–398 (III)

202. Zhang J, Bowes WA Jr, Fortney JA. Efficacy of external cephalic version: a review. Obstet Gynecol 1993;82:306–312 (III)

203. Newman RB, Peacock BS, VanDorsten JP, Hunt HH. Predicting success of external cephalic version. Am J Obstet Gynecol 1993;169:245–250 (II-3)

204. Van Veelan AJ, Van Cappellen AW, Flu PK, Straub MJ, Wallenburg HC. Effect of external cephalic version in late pregnancy on presentation at delivery: a randomized controlled trial. Br J Obstet Gynaecol 1989;96:916–921 (I)

205. Mahomed K, Seeras R, Coulson R. External cephalic version at term. A randomized controlled trial using tocolysis. Br J Obstet Gynaecol 1991;98:8–13 (I)

206. Brocks V, Philipsen T, Secher NJ. A randomized trial of external cephalic version with tocolysis in late pregnancy. Br J Obstet Gynaecol 1984;91:653–656 (I)

207. Goh JT, Johnson CM, Gregora MG. External cephalic version at term. Aust N Z J Obstet Gynaecol 1993;33:364–366 (III)

208. Dyson DC, Ferguson JE 2d, Hensleigh P. Antepartum external cephalic version under tocolysis. Obstet Gynecol 1986;67:63–68 (II-2)

209. Marchick R. Antepartum external cephalic version with tocolysis: a study of term singleton breech presentations. Am J Obstet Gynecol 1988;158:1339–1346 (II-3)

210. Cook HA. Experience with external cephalic version and selective vaginal breech delivery in private practice. Am J Obstet Gynecol 1993;168:1886–1890 (III)

211. Shalev E, Battino S, Giladi Y, Edelstein S. External cephalic version at term—using tocolysis. Acta Obstet Gynecol Scand 1993;72:455–457 (III)

212. Hellström AC, Nilsson B, Stange L, Nylund L. When does external cephalic version succeed? Acta Obstet Gynecol Scand 1990;69:281–285 (II-3)

213. American College of Obstetricians and Gynecologists. External cephalic version. ACOG Practice Bulletin 13. Washington: ACOG, 2000 (III)

214. Cheng M, Hannah M. Breech delivery at term: a critical review of the literature. Obstet Gynecol 1993;82:605–618 (III)

215. Donald WL, Barton JJ. Ultrasonography and external cephalic version at term. Am J Obstet Gynecol 1990;162:1542–1547 (III)

216. Morrison JC, Myatt RE, Martin JN Jr, Meeks GR, Martin RW, Bucovaz ET, et al. External cephalic version of the breech presentation under tocolysis. Am J Obstet Gynecol 1986;154:900–903 (II-3)

217. Hack M, Friedman H, Fanaroff AA. Outcomes of extremely low birth weight infants. Pediatrics 1996; 98:931–937 (II-2)

218. Ment LR, Oh W, Ehrenkranz RA, Philip AG, Duncan CC, Makuch RW. Antenatal steroids, delivery mode, and intraventricular hemorrhage in preterm infants. Am J Obstet Gynecol 1995;172: 795–800 (I)

219. Regenstein AC, Laros RK Jr, Wakeley A, Kitterman JA, Tooley WH. Mode of delivery in pregnancies complicated by preeclampsia with very low birth weight infants. J Perinatol 1995;15:2–6 (II-2)

220. Cibils LA, Karrison T, Brown L. Factors influencing neonatal outcomes in the very-low-birth-weight fetus (<1500 grams) with a breech presentation. Am J Obstet Gynecol 1994;171:35–42 (II-2)

221. Bethune M, Permezel M. The relationship between gestational age and the incidence of classical caesarean section. Aust N Z J Obstet Gynaecol 1997; 37:153–155 (II-3)

222. Bottoms SF, Paul RH, Iams JD, Mercer BM, Thom EA, Roberts JM, et al. Obstetric determinants of neonatal survival: influence of willingness to perform cesarean delivery on survival of extremely-low-birth-weight infants. National Institute of Child Health and Human Development Network of Maternal–Fetal Medicine Units. Am J Obstet Gynecol 1997;176: 960–966 (II-2)

223. Canadian Paediatric Society, Fetus and Newborn Committee, Society of Obstetricians and Gynaecologists of Canada, Maternal–Fetal Medicine Committee. Management of the woman with threatened birth of an infant of extremely low gestational age. CMAJ 1994;151:547–553 (III)

224. Penn ZJ, Steer PJ, Grant A. A multicentre randomised controlled trial comparing elective and selective caesarean section for the delivery of the preterm breech infant. Br J Obstet Gynaecol 1996; 103:684–689 (I)

225. Grant A, Penn ZJ, Steer PJ. Elective or selective caesarean delivery of the small baby? A systematic review of the controlled trials. Br J Obstet Gynaecol 1996;103:1197–1200 (MA)

226. American Society for Reproductive Medicine. Guidelines on number of embryos transferred. Available at: <http://www.asrm.org/current/practice/embryos.html>. Retrieved March 31, 1999 (III)

227. Chervenak FA, Johnson RE, Youcha S, Hobbins JC, Berkowitz RL. Intrapartum management of twin gestation. Obstet Gynecol 1985;64:119–124 (II-2)

228. Chervenak FA, Johnson RE, Berkowitz RL, Grannum P, Hobbins JC. Is routine cesarean section necessary for a vertex-breech and vertex-transverse twin gestation? Am J Obstet Gynecol 1984;148:1–5 (II-2)

229. Adam C, Allen AC, Baskett TF. Twin delivery: influence of presentation and method of delivery on the second twin. Am J Obstet Gynecol 1991;165: 23–27 (II-2)

230. Acker D, Lieberman M, Holbrook RH, James O, Phillippe M, Edelin KC. Delivery of the second twin. Obstet Gynecol 1982;59:710–711 (II-2)

231. Udom-Rice I, Skupski DW, Chervenak FA. Intrapartum management of multiple gestation. Semin Perinatol 1995;19:424–434 (III)

232. Gocke SE, Nageotte MP, Garite T, Towers CV, Dorchester W. Management of the nonvertex second twin: primary cesarean section, external version, or primary breech extraction. Am J Obstet Gynecol 1989;161:111–114 (II-2)

233. Greig PC, Veille JC, Morgan T, Henderson L. The effect of presentation and mode of delivery on neonatal outcome in the second twin. Am J Obstet Gynecol 1992;167:901–906 (II-2)

234. Davison L, Easterling TR, Jackson JC, Benedetti TJ. Breech extraction of low-birth-weight second twins: can cesarean section be justified? Am J Obstet Gynecol 1992:166:497–502 (II-2)

235. Bloomfield MM, Philipson EH. External cephalic version of twin A. Obstet Gynecol 1997;89:814–815 (III)

236. Fishman A, Grubb DK, Kovacs BW. Vaginal delivery of the nonvertex second twin. Am J Obstet Gynecol 1993;168:861–864 (II-2)

237. Leishman W. A system of midwifery, including the diseases of pregnancy and the puerperal state. 2nd American Edition. Philadelphia: Henry C. Lea, 1875; 473 (III)

238. Dennen EH. Forceps deliveries. Philadelphia, PA: F.A. Davis Company, 1955 (III)

239. American College of Obstetricians and Gynecologists. Delivery by vacuum extraction. ACOG Committee Opinion 208. Washington: ACOG, 1998 (III)

240. American College of Obstetricians and Gynecologists. Operative vaginal delivery. ACOG Practice Bulletin 17. Washington: ACOG, 2000 (III)

241. Hagadorn-Freathy AS, Yeomans ER, Hankins GD. Validation of the 1988 ACOG forceps classification system. Obstet Gynecol 1991;77:356–360 (II-3)

242. Hankins GD, Uckan E, Rowe TF, Collier S. Forceps and vacuum delivery: expectations of residency and fellowship training program directors. Am J Perinatol 1999;16:23–28 (II-3)

243. Carmona F, Martinez-Roman S, Manau D, Cararach V, Iglesias X. Immediate maternal and neonatal effects of low-forceps delivery according to the new criteria of the American College of Obstetricians and Gynecologists compared with spontaneous vaginal delivery in term pregnancies. Am J Obstet Gynecol 1995;173:55–59 (I)

244. Revah A, Ezra Y, Farine D, Ritchie K. Failed trial of vacuum or forceps—maternal and fetal outcome. Am J Obstet Gynecol 1997;176:200–204 (II-2)

245. Towner D, Castro MA, Eby-Wilkens E, Gilbert WM. Effect of mode of delivery in nulliparous women on neonatal intracranial injury. N Engl J Med 1999;341:1709–1714 (II-2)

246. Bofill JA, Rust OA, Perry KG, Roberts WE, Martin RW, Morrison JC. Operative vaginal delivery: a survey of fellows of ACOG. Obstet Gynecol 1996;88:1007–1010 (III)

247. Bofill JA, Rust OA, Perry KG Jr, Roberts WE, Martin RW, Morrison JC. Forceps and vacuum delivery: a survey of North American residency programs. Obstet Gynecol 1996;88:622–625 (II-3)

248. Hankins GD, Rowe TF. Operative vaginal delivery—year 2000. Am J Obstet Gynecol 1996;175:275–282 (III)

249. Notzon FC, Bergsjo P, Cole S, Irgens LM, Daltveit AK. International collaborative effort (ICE) on birth weight, plurality, perinatal, and infant mortality. IV. Differences in obstetric delivery practice: Norway, Scotland and the United States. Acta Obstet Gynecol Scand 1991;70:451–460 (III)

250. Zahniser SC, Kendrick JS, Franks AL, Saftlas AF. Trends in obstetric operative procedures, 1980 to 1987. Am J Public Health 1992;82:1340–1344 (II-3)

251. Lieberman E, Lang JM, Heffner LJ, Cohen A. Assessing the role of case mix in cesarean delivery rates. Obstet Gynecol 1998;92:1–7 (II-2)

252. Aron DC, Harper DL, Shepardson LB, Rosenthal GE. Impact of risk-adjusting cesarean delivery rates when reporting hospital performance. JAMA 1998;279:1968–1972(II-3)

253. Keeler EB, Park RE, Bell RM, Gifford DS, Keesey J. Adjusting cesarean delivery rates for case mix. Health Serv Res 1997;32:511–528 (III)

254. Cleary R, Beard RW, Chapple J, Coles J, Griffin M, Joffe M, et al. The standard primipara as a basis for inter-unit comparisons of maternity care. Br J Obstet Gynaecol 1996;103:223–229 (II-3)

255. Elliott JP, Russell MM, Dickason LA. The labor-adjusted cesarean section rate—a more informative method than the cesarean section "rate" for assessing a practitioner's labor and delivery skills. Am J Obstet Gynecol 1997;177:139–143 (III)

256. Main EK. Reducing cesarean birth rates with data-driven quality improvement activities. Pediatrics 1999;103:374–383 (II-3)

The MEDLINE database, the Cochrane Library, and ACOG's own internal resources and documents were used to conduct a literature search to locate relevant articles published between 1950 and 1999. The search was restricted to articles published in the English language. Priority was given to articles reporting results of original research, although review articles and commentaries also were consulted. Abstracts of research presented at symposia and scientific conferences were not considered adequate for inclusion in this document. Guidelines published by organizations or institutions such as the National Institutes of Health and the American College of Obstetricians and Gynecologists were reviewed, and additional studies were located by reviewing bibliographies of identified articles. When reliable research was not available, expert opinions from obstetrician–gynecologists were used.

Studies were reviewed and evaluated for quality according to the method outlined by the U.S. Preventive Services Task Force:

I Evidence obtained from at least one properly designed randomized controlled trial.

II-1 Evidence obtained from well-designed controlled trials without randomization.

II-2 Evidence obtained from well-designed cohort or case–control analytic studies, preferably from more than one center or research group.

II-3 Evidence obtained from multiple time series with or without the intervention. Dramatic results in uncontrolled experiments could also be regarded as this type of evidence.

III Opinions of respected authorities, based on clinical experience, descriptive studies, or reports of expert committees.

Appendix A. Nursing Data Base

Patient Identifier_____

Number of nurses who cared for patient _____

Nurse No.1 _____ (length of time)   _____ cm/dilatation (report as the range)

Nurse No.2 _____ (length of time)   _____ cm/dilatation (report as the range)

Nurse No.3 _____ (length of time)   _____ cm/dilatation (report as the range)

If more than 3 nurses list number _____

Amount of time patient received one-to-one nursing care _____

Did a doula attend the woman in labor and through birth? Yes _____   No _____

Estimate amount of time nurse is available to provide supportive care/comfort measures (time not related to technical or other interventions) _____

Appendix B. Cesarean Birth Evaluation Form

DATE COMPLETED	
PATIENT IDENTIFIER (OPTIONAL)	HOSPITAL IDENTIFIER
GESTATIONAL AGE: ___ ___ ___ / 7	PARITY _____ - _____ - _____ - _____

HISTORY
NO. PRIOR CESAREAN BIRTHS 0 1 2 3 4 MORE   PRIOR CLASSICAL? ☐ Y ☐ N   PRIOR VBAC? ☐ Y ☐ N
PRIOR SCARS (CIRCLE ALL THAT APPLY):
LOW TRANSVERSE   LOW VERTICAL   T-INCISION   CLASSICAL   MYOMECTOMY OR OTHER   UNKNOWN
INDICATION FOR ANY PRIOR CESAREAN DELIVERY (CIRCLE ALL THAT APPLY):
CPD/FAILURE   PRESENTATION/POSITION   FETAL INTOLERANCE TO LABOR   REPEAT   UNKNOWN   OTHER _____
NO. PRIOR VAGINAL BIRTHS   0 1 2 3 4 MORE   LARGEST PREVIOUS VAGINAL BIRTH _____LB   _____OZ   OR _____ G

CURRENT PREGNANCY
INDICATION FOR CURRENT CESAREAN (CIRCLE ALL THAT APPLY):
CPD/FAILURE   PRESENTATION/POSITION   FETAL INTOLERANCE TO LABOR   REPEAT   UNKNOWN   OTHER _____
TIME FROM ONSET OF LABOR TO CESAREAN: _____ HOURS (MAY BE 0)   INDUCTION? ☐ Y ☐ N
TIME FROM 5 CM CERVICAL DILATATION TO CESAREAN: _____ HOURS (MAY BE 0)

CIRCLE ALL THAT APPLY:	DIABETES HYPERTENSION
CIRCLE ALL THAT APPLY TO STATUS ON ADMISSION:	
FEVER ABRUPTION OLIGOHYDRAMNIOS IUGR POLYHYDRAMNIOS NONREASSURING FETAL EVALUATION	
PRESENTATION (CIRCLE ALL THAT APPLY):	VERTEX TRANSVERSE/OBLIQUE BREECH OTHER _____
IN CASE OF MULTIPLE BIRTH, PRESENTATION (CIRCLE ALL THAT APPLY):	VERTEX TRANSVERSE/OBLIQUE BREECH OTHER _____
POSITION IF VERTEX (CIRCLE 1):	NONVERTEX OA, LOA, OR ROA LOT OR ROT LOP, ROP, OR OP
LAST CERVICAL EXAMINATION PRIOR TO AROM (CIRCLE CLOSEST IN EACH CATEGORY, OR CHOOSE NO OR SROM)	
DILATATION (CM):	0 1 2 3 4 5 6 7 8 9 10
EFFACEMENT (%):	0 25 50 75 100
STATION: FLOATING   -3   -2   -1   0   +1   +2   +3 STATION
NO OR SROM	

51

CURRENT PREGNANCY (CONTINUED)

LAST CERVICAL EXAMINATION PRIOR TO EPIDURAL (CIRCLE CLOSEST IN EACH CATEGORY, OR MARK NO EPIDURAL)

DILATATION (CM):	0 1 2 3 4 5 6 7 8 9 10
EFFACEMENT (%):	0 25 50 75 100
STATION: FLOATING   −3   −2   −1   0   +1   +2   +3 STATION

NO EPIDURAL

LAST CERVICAL EXAMINATION PRIOR TO CESAREAN (CIRCLE CLOSEST IN EACH CATEGORY, OR MARK NOT EXAMINED)

DILATATION (CM):	0 1 2 3 4 5 6 7 8 9 10
EFFACEMENT (%):	0 25 50 75 100
STATION: FLOATING   −3   −2   −1   0   +1   +2   +3 STATION

NOT EXAMINED

TIME FROM ROM TO CESAREAN: _____ HOURS (IF DAYS OR WEEKS, CONVERT TO HOURS) (MAY BE ZERO)

TIME MAKING PROGRESS AT = 1 CM/HR PRIOR TO CESAREAN: _____ HOURS (MAY BE 0)

INDICATION FOR INDUCTION:

PROM   PREECLAMPSIA   ELECTIVE   POSTDATES   SUSPECTED MACROSOMIA   PLANNED REPEAT   OTHER INDICATION _____

TIME FROM ONSET OXYTOCIN TO CESAREAN: _____ HOURS (MAY BE 0)

FETAL/NEONATAL DATA

ESTIMATED FETAL WEIGHT: _____

FETAL HEART RATE DESCRIPTION PRIOR TO CESAREAN (CIRCLE ONE ON EACH LINE):

VARIABILITY:	NORMAL/INCREASED	DECREASED	NONE	NOT DESCRIBED
DECELERATIONS:	DEEP VARIABLES	LATES/LATE COMPONENT	OTHER	NOT DESCRIBED
BASELINE RATE: ____/MIN	BRACHYCARDIA	TACHYCARDIA	NORMAL	NOT DESCRIBED
LAST SCALP STIMULATION:	REASSURING	NONREASSURING	NOT DONE	
LAST ACOUSTIC STIMULATION:	REASSURING	NONREASSURING	NOT DONE	

LAST SCALP pH (0.00 IF NOT DONE): _____

BIRTHWEIGHT (0 IF NOT RECORDED): _____ _____ _____ _____   IF A MULTIPLE GESTATION, N=_____

APGARS: ____ /____ /____   ____ /____ /____   ____ /____ /____   ____ /____ /____

CORD GASES:

ARTERY pH _____ P_{CO_2} ____ P_{O_2} ____ BE ____

VEIN pH ____ P_{CO_2} ____ P_{O_2} ____ BE ____

UNKNOWN VESSEL

BABY TO: ICN/SPECIAL CARE   FULL TERM   MOTHER'S ROOM   MORGUE

(DATA GATHERER)	(PLEASE PRINT NAME)

Appendix C. Sample Calculations for Case-Mix Adjustment Using Standardization

A single institution's unadjusted cesarean delivery rates for hospital-based practices (24.4%) and community-based practices (21.5%) are studied to illustrate the use of standardization for case-mix adjustment of cesarean delivery rates. A standardized rate of cesarean delivery for the hospital-based practice was calculated using the community-based practitioners' case mix as the standard population. The resulting standardized rate indicates what the cesarean delivery rate for the hospital-based practice would be if they saw the same patients as the community-based practitioners. The following steps were performed to make the adjustment:

1. Women were classified into one of the parity and obstetric condition subgroups (nulliparous women, multiparous women without previous cesarean delivery, multiparous women with previous cesarean delivery, multiple pregnancy, breech presentation, preterm delivery, medical condition precluding a trial of labor, term singleton fetus with cephalic presentation with specified medical condition, or term singleton fetus with cephalic presentation without specified medical condition) using the answers to the eight yes or no questions in the box.

2. The cesarean delivery rate for each of the parity and obstetric condition subgroups for the hospital practice was determined (Table 1).

3. Each subgroup's percentage of the standard population (community-based practice) was determined (Table 1).

4. The hospital cesarean delivery rate for each subgroup was multiplied by the percentage of women in that subgroup in the community-based practice. The products from the multiplication for each subgroup were totaled to obtain the standardized cesarean delivery rate.

The unadjusted rate for the hospital-based practice was substantially higher than the rate for community-

---

Classification Form to Implement Standardization of Cesarean Delivery Rates

1. Was the woman nulliparous or multiparous?
2. If the woman was multiparous, did she have a previous cesarean delivery?
3. Was this a multiple pregnancy?
4. Was the fetus in a breech presentation or transverse lie?
5. Was the fetus younger than 36 weeks of gestation?
6. Was there a medical condition precluding a trial of labor (as determined by the physician)?
7. Were any of the following conditions present (hypertension, diabetes, birth $\geq$ 4,500 g, or one of the following at admission: fever $\geq$100.4°F, placental abruption, oligohydramnios, polyhydramnios, intrauterine growth restriction, nonreassuring fetal condition)?
8. Was a cesarean delivery performed?

Lieberman E, Lang JM, Heffner LJ, Cohen A. Assessing the role of case mix in cesarean delivery rates. Obstet Gynecol 1998;92:1–7

---

based practitioners (24.4% versus 21.5%). The standardized rate indicates, however, that if the hospital-based practice's patient mix were the same as that seen by community-based practitioners, the hospital-based practice would have a cesarean delivery rate of 20.1%, not much different from the community-based practitioner's cesarean delivery rate of 21.5% (1).

1. Lieberman E, Lang JM, Heffner LJ, Cohen A. Assessing the role of case mix in cesarean delivery rates. Obstet Gynecol 1998;92:1–7

Table 1. Data and Calculations for Determination of the Standardized Cesarean Delivery Rate for Hospital-Based Practitioners Using Community-Based Practices as the Standard Population*

Obstetric Condition Category	Nulliparous Women		Multiparous Women Without Previous Cesarean Delivery		Multiparous Women with Previous Cesarean Delivery	
	Hospital-Based Cesarean Delivery Rate (%)	Proportion of Community-Based Practices	Hospital-Based Cesarean Delivery Rate (%)	Proportion of Community-Based Practices	Hospital-Based Cesarean Delivery Rate (%)	Proportion of Community-Based Practices
Multiple pregnancy	66.0	.013	60.9	.008	100.0	.002
Breech presentation or transverse lie	96.2	.022	83.8	.009	100.0	.007
Preterm delivery	27.2	.018	21.7	.007	61.9	.005
No trial of labor	100.0	.010	100.0	.004	100.0	.016
≥36 weeks of gestation with medical risk	23.7	.089	8.3	.044	48.3	.012
≥36 weeks of gestation without medical risk	12.1	.337	3.1	.325	39.0	.073

* Calculations for determining the standardized rate of cesarean delivery for the hospital-based group:
0.013 (66.0) + 0.022 (96.2) + 0.018 (27.2) + 0.010 (100.0) + 0.089 (23.7) + 0.337 (12.1) +
0.008 (60.9) + 0.009 (83.8) +0.007 (21.7) + 0.004 (100.0) + 0.044 (8.3) + 0.325 (3.1) +
0.002 (100.0) + 0.007 (100.0) + 0.005 (61.9) + 0.016 (100.0) +0.012 (48.3) + 0.073 (39.0)
= 20.1% standardized rate
Lieberman E, Lang JM, Heffner LJ, Cohen A. Assessing the role of case mix in cesarean delivery rates. Obstet Gynecol 1998;92:1–7

Index